MR Angiography Applications in Pediatric Intracranial Vascular Lesions

MR ANGIOGRAPHY APPLICATIONS IN PEDIATRIC INTRACRANIAL VASCULAR LESIONS

R. Nuri Sener, M.D.
Professor of Radiology
Ege University Hospital
Department of Radiology
Bornova, Izmir, Turkey

formerly
Research Fellow at the University of Texas
Health Science Center
Department of Radiology, Neuroradiology Section
San Antonio, Texas, U.S.A.

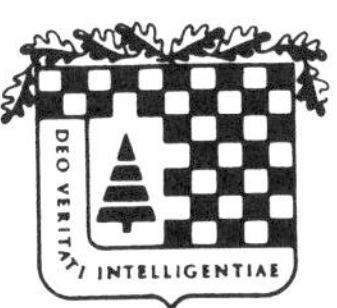

WARREN H. GREEN, INC,
St. Louis, Missouri, U.S.A.

Published by

WARREN H. GREEN, INC.
8356 Olive Boulevard
St. Louis, Missouri 63132, U.S.A.

ISBN No. 0-87527-526-5

Sener, R. Nuri

Printed in the United States of America

To Özge Özgürler

Foreword

It is my pleasure to write the foreword to this monograph, *MR Angiography Applications in Pediatric Intracranial Vascular Lesions*, by R. Nuri Sener. Historically, beginning with conventional radiographic studies, cranial angiography has gone through progressive technical advancements. Digital subtraction angiography and computed tomographic angiography have both made subsequent contributions to the diagnosis of intracranial disease. However, these modalities require the use of intervascular contrast agents and are invasive to various degrees. MR angiography, on the other hand, is capable of visualizing the major arteries and veins of the cranium noninvasively and without the need of injected contrast agents. This is especially important in the imaging analysis of pediatric cranial disease, because invasive angiography in these patients is technically difficult and carries a real risk of serious complications.

This monograph provides an excellent review of many of the common pathologic conditions that may affect the cranial vasculature in the pediatric population. The more rare examples are significant as they point out the potential possibilities of MR angiography in the diagnosis of cranial vascular disease. Overall, Dr. Sener has successfully produced a concise overview of the applications of this exciting new technique and impresses upon us the promising future of MR angiography.

J. Randy Jinkins, M.D.
Director of Neuroradiology
University of Texas Health Sciences Center
7703 F. Curl Drive
San Antonio, Texas 782840-7800

CONTENTS

MR Angiography Applications in Pediatric Intracranial Vascular Lesions

MR Angiography Applications in Pediatric Intracranial Vascular Lesions

Magnetic resonance (MR) imaging has become a reliable, noninvasive method for detecting intracranial vascular lesions such as vascular malformations, aneurysms, occlusions, and some others. MR angiography (MRA), although still is inferior to conventional and digital subtraction angiography, is a promising noninvasive method of examination. The present booklet covers not only the relatively common or commonly studied vascular lesions, but also a number of unusual lesions, and unusual applications of MRA in intracranial vascular abnormalities in pediatric patients.

Technical considerations

Current clinical application of intracranial MRA is usually based on 3-dimensional time-of-flight (3D-TOF) and 3-dimensional phase-contrast (3D-PC) methods for projection arteriograms, and on a 2-dimensional time-of-flight (2D-TOF) method for projection venograms. These techniques are available in most of the recent MR units (including the 0.5T unit we used). There are a number of recent advances in MRA techniques usually installed on more sophisticated units, such as 3D-multivolume MRA, magnitude contrast MRA, turbo MRA, black blood imaging, breath-hold techniques and some others. Advantages of the 3D-PC technique include its sensitivity to slow flow (low flow velocity can be utilized for demonstration of slowly flowing vessels), and good background suppression. Its limitations are relatively long acquisition time and sensitivity to pulsatile flow. 3D-TOF technique has a relatively short acquisition time, and good isotopic resolution, however, it is limited by progressive spin saturation and by its T1 sensitivity (fat, blood products and contrast medium). 2D-TOF technique is sensitive to flow, and it is limited by in-plane saturation of spins. Utilization of different techniques in different planes in the particular subject usually can produce satisfactory MRA images [Charakes et al. (1991), Creasy et al. (1990), Davis et al. (1994), Dumoulin et al. (1989), Huston and Ehman (1993), Levin and Laub (1991), Mattle et al. (1991)].

MR imaging examinations of pediatric patients in this booklet were performed at 0.5 Tesla using the GE Vectra (*General Electric, USA*). They included the conventional spin-echo and gradient recalled-echo (T1-weighted), and inversion recovery (T1-weighted) pulse sequences, and MR angiography (MRA), usually performed at the same session. MRA was the 2D-TOF, and 3D-PC (applied at the region of centrum semiovale in an axial plane and with a slow flow velocity, i.e. 6-20 cm/sec) techniques for projection MR venograms. Both will be referred to as MR angiography (MRA) throughout the text.

Details of MRA examinations were as follows:

(a) The parameters for 3D-TOF MRA usually were: TR=60ms, TE=10ms, Flip angle=25 degrees, Matrix=128x224, NEX=1, FOV=20, and Slice thickness=1mm, Depth matrix=48mm, Slab thickness=48mm (variable). Flow compensation, rectangular pixel, and half-echo were utilized.

(b) The parameters for 3D-PC MRA usually were: TR=32ms (variable), TE=13ms (variable), Flip angle=20 degrees, Flow-velocity (variable, based on TR values) = 6-40cm/sec, Matrix=128x256, FOV=25, Slice spacing=0mm, and Slice thickness=1.25mm, Depth matrix=48mm, Slab thickness=60mm (variable). Rectangular pixel was utilized, and

(c) The parameters for 2D-TOF MRA usually were: TR=60ms, TE=10ms, Flip angle=90 degrees, Matrix=128x256, NEX=1, FOV=20, Slice spacing=0mm Slice thickness=4mm. Presaturation (towards feet), flow compensation, and half-echo were utilized.

Maximum intensity projections (MIP) were obtained either from the whole slab or by dividing it usually by 2 or sometimes by 3, as required.

Intracranial Vascular Lesions in Pediatric Patients

Intracranial vascular lesions diseases comprise a wide variety of lesions including hypoxic-ischemic encephalopathy, hemorrhage, arteritis and arteriopathy, arterial and venous infarction, and vascular lesions such as malformations and aneurysms. Conventional MR imaging has been a sensitive modality in the evaluation of most of these. In the recent years MRA emerges as a promising noninvasive method of examination. We have included MRA applications in various intracranial vascular lesions in 40 patients.

Arteriovenous malformation

It has been considered that arteriovenous malformations are the most common type of congenital vascular malformations in the general population. They occur throughout the central nervous system, and are characterized by a direct communication between the arterial and venous circulations without an intervening capillary bed. They consist of pial (parenchymal), dural, and mixed (pial-dural) malformations. About half of these patients experience intracranial hemorrhage, and the common age at presentation is between 20 and 40 years, although it an be seen anytime [Huston et al. (1991), Nussel et al. (1991), Osborn (1994)]. Different types of arteriovenous malformations are illustrated in Figures 1-7, 14, and 15.

Aneurysm

In general, it is believed that fusiform aneurysms are secondary to atherosclerosis, and saccular (berry) aneurysms are congenital. Berry aneurysms most frequently involve the carotid circulation. And, a small number of aneurysms are caused by micotic infection, trauma or neoplasms [Huston et al. (1991), Osborn (1994), Ross et al. (1990)]. Although, relatively larger unruptured aneurysms (i.e. 6 mm in diameter or larger) can usually be easily identified on spin-echo MR imaging, and on 3D-PC MRA and 3D-TOF MRA (detection rate = 100%), recent studies at 1.5 Tesla indicated that smaller lesion may escape detection especially on 3D-PC MRA, because of its sensitivity to pulsatile flow [Araki et al. (1994), Huston et al. (1994)]. An aneurysm associated with a mixed arteriovenous malformation is shown in Figure 8. Also, a patient whose 8-mm aneurysm was easily shown on spin-echo MR imaging, and on 3D-TOF MRA, but not on 3D-PC MRA is illustrated (Figure 9).

Venous malformation

Venous malformations (angiomas) represent vascular lesions involving only the venous side of the circulation, and no abnormal arterial component is present. They are usually intraparenchymal. They can be seen at any age, often as an incidental finding on imaging studies (CT and MR imaging). They are often asymptomatic. Occasionally they can bleed and may cause seizures [Osborn (1994)]. Although, a venous malformation can readily be detected on spin-echo or gradient recalled-echo images, their demonstration by MR angiography may be problematic. They may be seen on a 2D-TOF MRA, but a 3D-TOF MRA is usually negative. A 3D-PC MRA with a low flow velocity (i.e. 6cm/sec) is usually required for their demonstration [Damiano et al.(1994), Ostertun and Solymosi (1993)]. An example of the condition is included studied by 3D-PC MRA with a low flow velocity (Figure 10). A pitfall of 3D-PC MRA (with high flow velocity) is shown in Figure 11.

Vein of Galen malformation

Vein of Galen malformation is a rare congenital anomaly believed to result from a lack of regression of the primitive prosencephalic vein of Markowski. It is characterized by abnormal connections (via either a direct arteriovenous fistula or via a nidus of arteriovenous malformation) between the intracranial arteries and the vein of Galen. In most cases there is a venous outflow restriction in the straight sinus or other dural sinuses [Lasjaunas et al. (1991), Seidenwurm et al. (1991)]. MRA appears to be a promising modality as acquisition of hemodynamic information by MRA regarding the extent of the malformation is comparable to that obtained from conventional angiography, such as distinction of a arteriovenous fistula from arteriovenous malformation supplying the galenic malformation, and demonstration of the sites of venous outflow restriction [Sener (1997)]. These data would enable direct performance of therapeutic angiography (avoiding diagnostic angiography) with minimum contrast load to the patient. Herein MRA of two patients are included with galenic malformations (Figures 12 and 13).

Varix of the dural sinuses associated with arteriovenous malformations and other abnormalities

Varix of the torcula and ectatic dural sinuses associated with mixed arteriovenous malformations and fistulae, is a rare condition. Dural arteriovenous malformations and fistulae are associated with a network of dural arteries and fistulae and dilated draining veins and dural sinuses. The etiology of the condition has usually been attributed to dural sinus thrombosis and recanalization, hence an acquired condition. These patients usually present between the ages 40 and 60 years. In contrast to this acquired type, rarely some congenital types may occur [ApSimon et al. (1993), Chen et al. (1992)]. Varix of the torcula and ectatic dural sinuses associated with mixed arteriovenous malformations and fistulae, is probably a congenital condition. A few similar cases associated with a large torcular varix have previously been reported by conventional angiography [ApSimon et al. (1993)]. We illustrate MRA findings in a 4.5-year-old patient with a varix of the torcula and dural sinuses associated with mixed arteriovenous malformations (Figure 14). Another patient with a varix of the dural sinus, parenchymal arteriovenous malformation, mineralizing microangiopathy, and an abnormal cerebellum is shown in Figure 15.

Dural sinus thrombosis

Dural sinus thrombosis results from meningitis, sepsis, or infections of contiguous sites, especially if the patient is dehydrated. It can be associated with either bland or hemorrhagic infarcts due to occlusion of the cortical veins. The superior sagittal sinus is the most commonly occluded dural sinus, followed by the transverse, sigmoid, and cavernous sinuses. Thombosis may extend to the jugular veins. In dural sinus thrombosis, there usually is a broad spectrum of nonspecific symptoms and clinical findings. Also, some normal conditions as well as some artifacts on CT and MR imaging may cause some confusion [Osborn (1994)]. Therefore, care should be exercised while either in diagnosing or excluding the condition. We present two patients, one with true dural sinus thrombosis and hemorrhagic infarctions (Figure 16), and the other with a false thrombosis verified utilizing a variety of diagnostic modalities (Figure 17). It has been cited that there is a high variation in the velocity of blood flow in the dural sinuses, ranging from approximately 20 to 45 cm/sec [Vogl et al. (1994)]. A more slow flow within a vessel may mimic a dural sinus thrombosis, as shown in our patient (Figure 17). It is generally accepted that a 2D-TOF MRA obtained in multiple projections is a reliable method for investigation of flow in dural sinuses [Vogl et al. (1994)]. We have demonstrated that a 3D-PC MRA obtained by a very low velocity encoding (i.e. 7cm/sec) may also be useful for this purpose (Figure 17).

Vertebrobasilar dissection

Dissection of the carotid and vertebral arteries may occur after major trauma, spontaneously or after trivial injury. The condition is most commonly seen in persons in the third to fifth decade, however, no age group is spared. Dissection of the vertebral artery occurs less frequently than dissection of the internal carotid artery. Most of the patients recover fully unless frank subarachnoid hemorrhage is associated with the condition. Prompt anticoagulation therapy can prevent infarctions provided that such contraindications as subarachnoid hemorrhage or large infarctions are not present [Bui et al.(1993), Klufas et al. (1995)].

We illustrate a patient with traumatic dissection of the left vertebral artery which extended to the basilar artery (Figure 18).

Absence of the vertebral artery

It is known that a hypoplastic vertebral artery is common in up to 40% of normal conventional angiograms. Duplication, and fenestration of the vertebral artery occasionally occurs [Osborn, (1994)]. Total absence of a vertebral artery is a rare condition, and its diagnosis by MRA is not yet reliable, and requires conventional angiography including an arch aortography and subclavian angiography. We studied a patient with a known absence of the right vertebral artery (shown by conventional angiography), by coronal 3D-PC MRA (Figure 19).

Intracranial vasculitis

Primary cerebral arteritis is a rare disease of unknown cause. The disease commonly affects the small leptomeningeal vessels. However, any vessel including the large intracranial arteries can be involved. Primary cerebral arteritis is characterized by neurologic dysfunction that remains unexplained after thorough clinical, laboratory, neurologic, and radiologic investigation, provided that no disease process causing systemic vasculitis is evident. Therefore its diagnosis is frequently one of exclusion. With respect to radiologic findings, usually there are multiple small foci of infarction or hemorrhage. The lesions have previously been demonstrated on conventional MR imaging and angiographic studies. Especially, multiple punctate areas of contrast-enhancement on MR imaging has been shown. Conventional angiography usually shows stenosis of the affected vessels [Greenan et al. (1992) Harris et al. (1994), Schoemaker et al. (1994)]. We illustrate a patient who had consistent clinicoradiologic findings with primary cerebral arteritis. Postcontrast T1-weighted MR images, in particular, were suggestive of the lesion. MR angiography showed multiple collateral vessels in the basal ganglia suggesting arteritis, which was confirmed by conventional angiography (Figure 20). Another patient with vasculitis involving the right internal carotid artery is shown in Figure 21.

Moyamoya disease

Moyamoya disease represents a progressive occlusive arteriopathy of childhood or adolescence. Repeated ischemic episodes are common. Progressive stenosis of the supraclinoid internal carotid artery and proximal anterior and middle cerebral arteries is seen. Involvement is frequently bilateral. Multiple, extensive parenchymal, leptomeningeal, and transdural collateral vessels develop. Large vessel occlusions as well as major collateral flow patterns can be demonstrated by MRA [Yamada et al. (1992)]. We illustrate a patient with moyamoya disease associated with unilateral changes (Figure 22). This patient had an operation in order to increase the arterial flow to the right hemisphere (an encephalodural arteriomyosynangiosis was performed). A follow-up MRA study revealed apparent improvement of the vascular stenosis (Figure 23).

Leukemic vasculopathy

In leukemia, meningitis is an occasional intracranial manifestation. Rarely, intracranial masses may occur, which are called "chloromas." The presence of these are usually confined to myelocytic leukemia [Sze et al. (1989), Leonard and Mamorian (1989)]. We present a patient with acute lymphoblastic leukemia with spastic narrowing of the middle cerebral arteries (vasculopathy) associated with parenchymal ischemic lesions, and speculate that the spasm of these arteries is a reactional phenomenon to the hematologic changes associated with leukemia [Sener (1995)] (Figure 24).

Spontaneous carotid-cavernous fistula

Carotid-cavernous fistulas most often result from trauma. Less commonly, a spontaneous type of carotid-cavernous fistula may occur in primarily middle aged woman. There usually a single direct communication between the internal carotid artery and cavernous sinus. Drainage most commonly occurs via the ipsilateral superior opthalmic vein, although a bilateral drainage is not infrequent, and a contralateral drainage can rarely occur [Barkovich (1995), Chen et al. (1992)]. Hemophiliac patients may be predicted to develop spontaneous carotid-cavernous fistulas, as in the patient with factor VIII deficiency we illustrate (Figure 25).

Neuronal migrational disorders

It is known that neuronal migrational disorders can be associated with abnormal venous drainage. This has been shown in the past with conventional MR imaging and angiography [Barkovich (1988)]. Abnormal venous drainage is especially common in regions of polymicrogyria, a disorder of neuronal migration and sulcation, where there is a large infolding of thickened cortex. Such vessels show no arteriovenous shunting or no tangles of vessels, and should not be misinterpreted as vascular malformations [Barkovich (1995)]. They can be demonstrated by MRA [Sener (1995)]. We illustrate vascular changes in several patients with polymicrogyria by MRA (Figures 28-30). The appearance of the normal cortical veins on 3D-PC MRA, and on 3D-TOF MRA (in an axial slab centered to the centrum semiovale) is included for comparison (Figures 26, 27).

Periventricular leukomalacia

Periventricular leukomalacia is an ischemic lesion of the periventricular white matter which is considered to result from diminished cerebral perfusion. It eventually leads to a localized loss of cerebral volume associated with gliosis [Truwit et al. (1992)]. In a recent study (Sener (1997)] we usually noted a single prominent abnormal vein within the affected hemisphere. Although the reason for this appears to be unclear, we speculate that during the perinatal ischemic episode and subsequent volume loss and gliosis, most of the cortical veins become collapsed (and obstructed) in the affected region, leaving behind a few normal ones, and consequently one (or more) of which becomes slightly thickened, and elongated to enable effective venous drainage from the region. Such abnormal vessels should not be misinterpreted as vascular malformations. There patients with periventricular leukomalacia with such vessels are illustrated (Figures 31-33) (compare with Figures 26, 27). Also, thinned middle cerebral arteries in another patient with diffuse periventricular leukomalacia is demonstrated by MRA (Figure 34), and the MRA of normal middle cerebral arteries is included for comparison (Figure 35).

Arachnoid cyst

Arachnoid cysts are congenital or acquired CSF-filled collections, more than half of which occur in the middle cranial fossa, and the remaining are located in the suprasellar and quadrigeminal regions, or in the posterior fossa, or over the frontal convexities. Bilateral middle cranial fossa cysts are very rare [Robertson et al. (1989), Wolpert and Barnes (1992)]. A temporal region arachnoid cyst displacing the middle cerebral artery is illustrated by MRA (Figure 36). Another patient with an unusual trilobated arachnoid cyst which occupied the middle cranial fossae and the suprasellar region associated with a retroclival extension is illustrated. MRA provided optimal demonstration of the gross vascular displacement (Figure 37).

Cavernous angioma

The MR imaging features of cavernous angiomas are usually characteristic especially when a central core of hyperintensity (methemoglobin) is surrounded by a ring of hypointensity (hemosiderin), which is best appreciated on spin-echo T2-weighted MR images. Sometimes the entire lesion may be hypointense due to the presence of chronic hemorrhagic products (hemosiderin) [Gomori et al. (1986)].

Some authors [Huston (1993)] commented that the appearance of a cavernous angioma on TOF angiography could reflect T1-shortening caused by subacute hemorrhagic products (methemoglobin), but not the lesion itself, a known drawback of that technique. In the patient we illustrate, however, the lesion was hypointense on the 2D-TOF MRA while it was hyperintense on 3D-TOF MRA. Also, the lesion was hypointense both on T1W and T2W images (no T1-shortening). We consider the discrepancy between the two TOF angiograms, and lack of T1-shortening, in favor of direct visualization of the cavernous angioma itself on the 3D-TOF MRA. Gradient recalled-echo images excluded an arteriovenous malformation (Figure 38).

Fibrous dysplasia

Fibrous dysplasia is a developmental osseous disorder in which cancellous bone is replaced with fibrous tissue resulting in expansion of the bone. The disease presents in either a monostotic or a polyostotic form. The polyostotic form of the condition, when associated with skin pigmentation and endocrine abnormalities leading to accelerated maturation and sexual prematurity, is known as the McCune-Albright syndrome. Cranial involvement is seen in most of these patients.

We studied a patient with an extensive cranial involvement with polyostotic fibrous dysplasia by MRA, which showed abnormal extracranial and transcranial vessels. [Sener (1997)] (Figure 39).

Intracranial tumors and mass lesions

MRA mainly provides information on vascular displacement, distortion, narrowing or occlusion caused by intracranial tumors. Recent advances in MRA techniques installed on more sophisticated units, and use of contrast medium may provide further data on vascularization patterns of different tumor types. We illustrate four patients with intracranial mass lesions; three with tumors (Figures 40-42), and one with fibrous dysplasia of the clivus (Figure 43) on MRA.

Intracerebral hemorrhage

Intracerebral hemorrhage may be caused by hypertension, stroke, trauma, tumors, perinatal causes, aneurysms, vascular malformations, infarction, inflammatory disease, blood dyscrasia and some others [Osborn (1994)]. The expected role of MRA is to noninvasively discriminate lesions secondary to aneurysms, vascular malformations from others, however, at the present time conventional angiography is mandatory in any equivocal condition. We illustrate a patient with intracerebral hemorrhage by MRA with a comparison of the 3D-PC MRA, and 3D-TOF MRA (Figure 44).

SUMMARY

MRA is a noninvasive, effective screening technique for 3-dimensional visualization of a wide range of intracranial vascular lesions in pediatric patients. The present booklet covers not only the relatively common or commonly studied vascular lesions, but also a number of unusual lesions, and unusual applications of MRA in abnormalities such as intracranial vasculitis, neuronal migrational disorders, periventricular leukomalacia, and fibrous dysplasia. The 3D-TOF and 3D-PC MRA techniques produce projection MR arteriograms, and the 2D-TOF and 3D-PC techniques produce projection MR venograms. It is particularly noted that the 3D-PC technique applied at the region of centrum semiovale in an axial plane and with a slow flow velocity (i.e. 6-20 cm/sec) can produce good projection MR venograms for evaluation of neuronal migrational disorders and periventricular leukomalacia, and other vascular lesions at this region with slow flowing vessels. It is concluded that MR angiography is a noninvasive, effective screening technique for 3-dimensional visualization of a wide range of intracranial vascular lesions in pediatric patients.

FIGURES

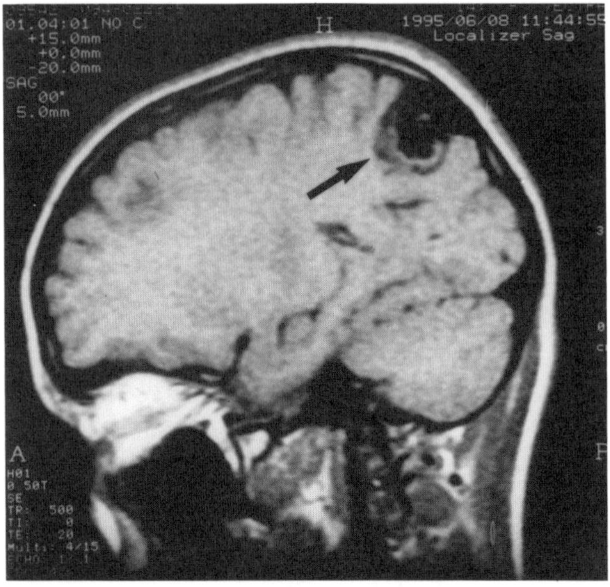

1a

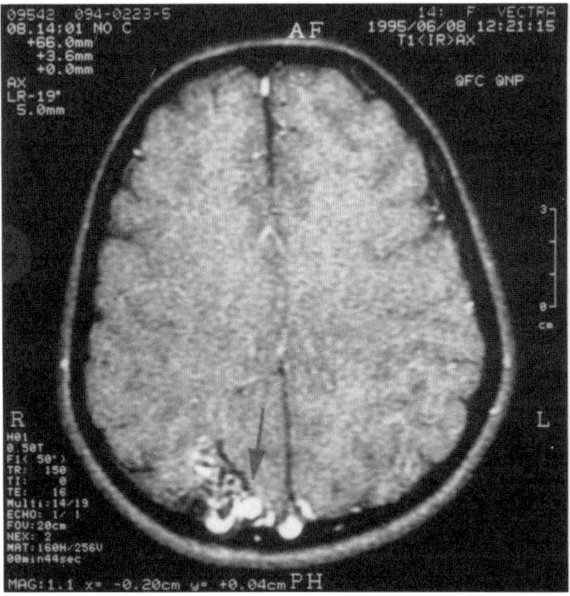

1b

Fig.1 *a-e. Arteriovenous malformation.* 14-year-old girl. *a,* sagittal spin-echo T1-weighted (T1W); *b,* axial gradient-recalled echo T1-weighted (GRE T1W) MR images; *c,* coronal 3-dimensional phase-contrast MR angiography (3D-PC MRA); *d,* sagittal 3D-PC MR; and *e,* axial 3-dimensional time-of-flight MR angiography (3D-TOF MRA).

A right parietal, parenchymal arteriovenous malformation is seen (arrows, *a-e*) supplied by the posterior parietal branch of the middle cerebral artery (arrowheads, *c-e*), and draining to the superior sagittal sinus.

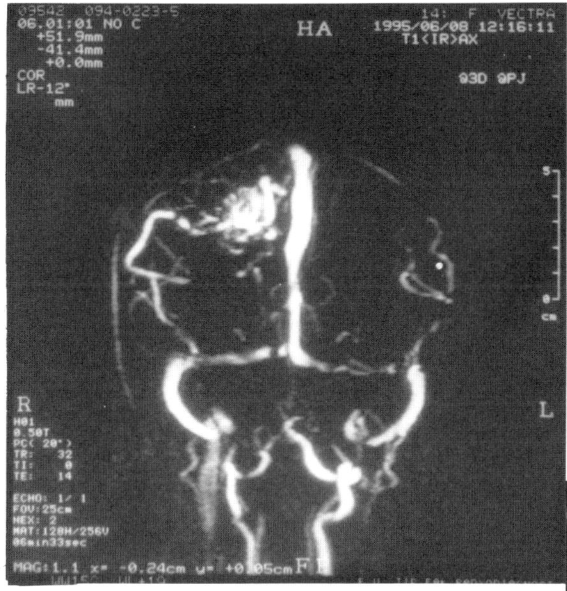

1c

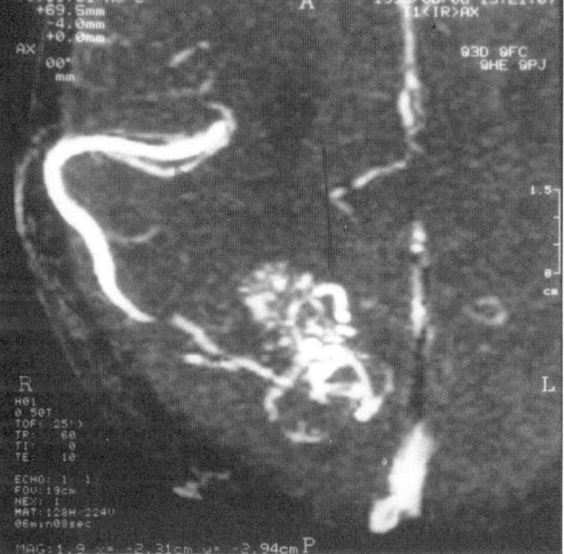

1e

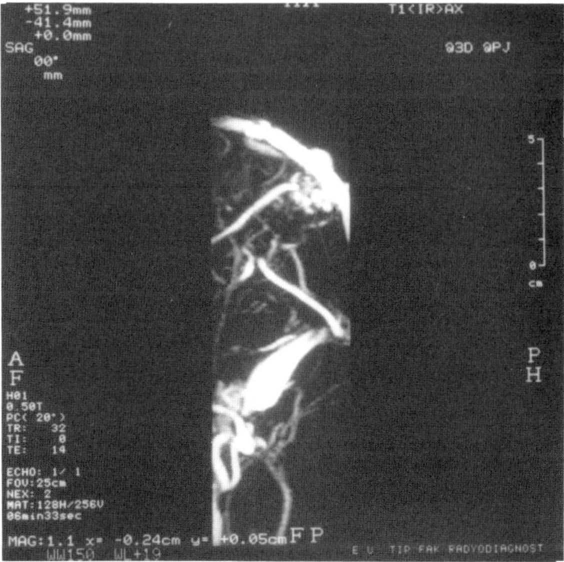

1d

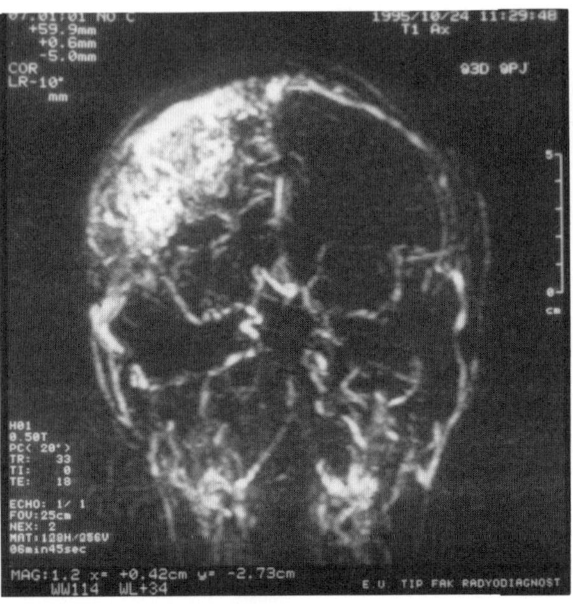

2a

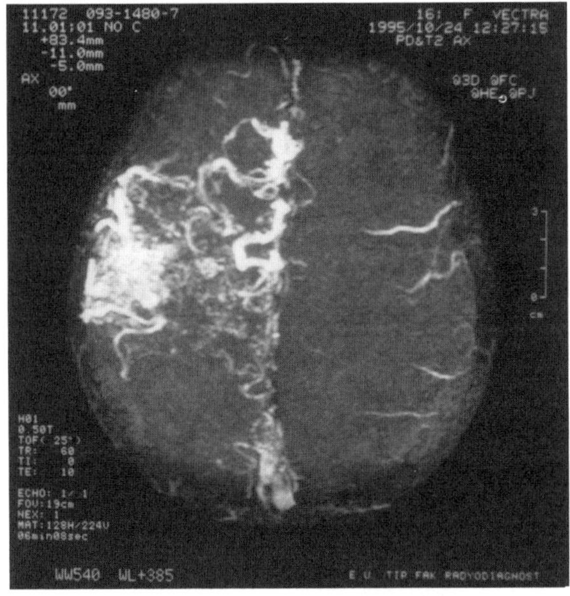

2b

Fig. 2 *a,b*. *Arteriovenous malformation*. 16-year-old girl. *a,* coronal 3D-PC MRA; and *b,* axial 3D-TOF MRA. An extensive, parenchymal arteriovenous malformation is seen involving the right hemisphere, supplied by the branches of the middle and anterior cerebral arteries (arrows, *a,b*), and draining to the superior sagittal and transverse sinuses.

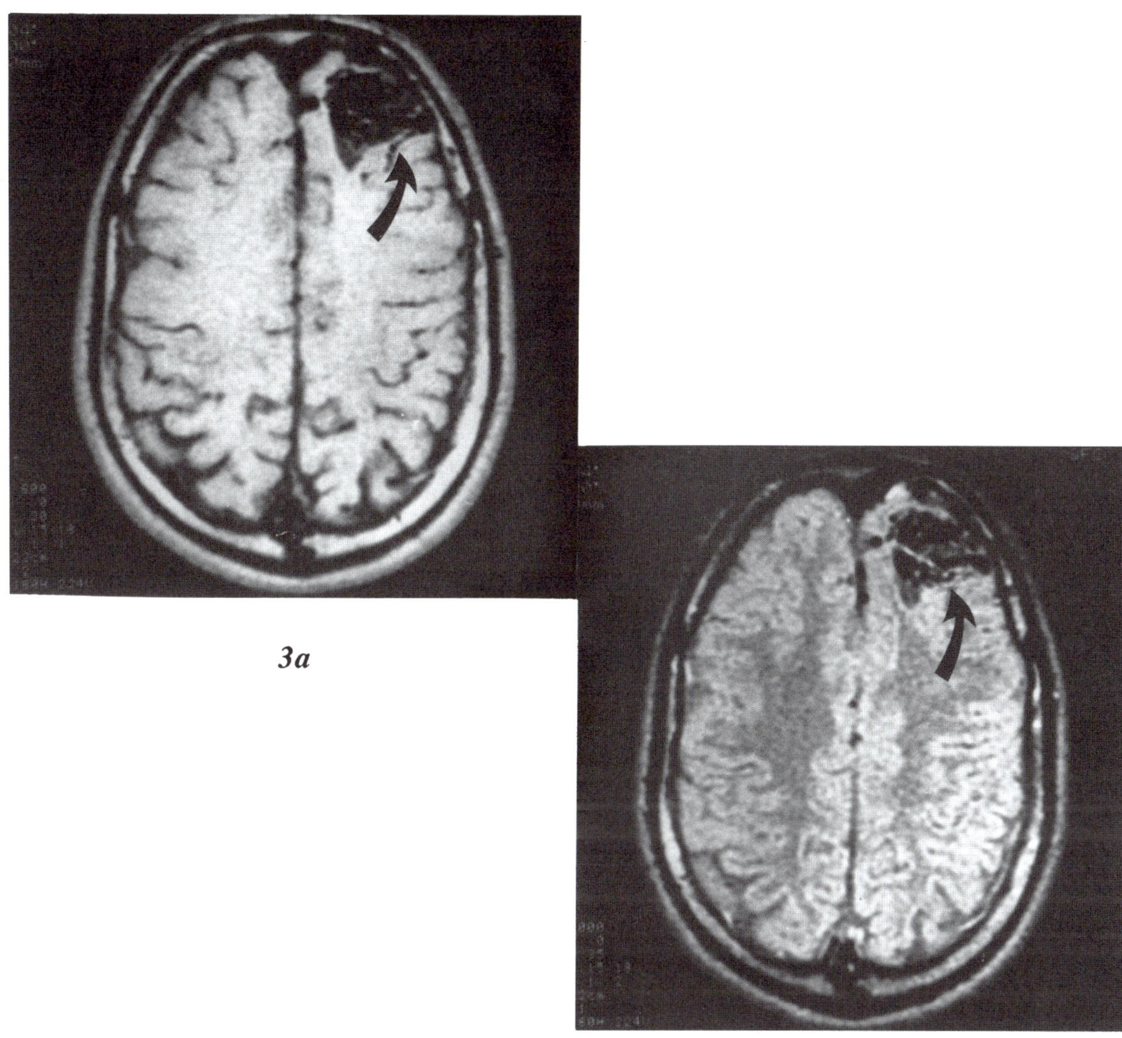

3a

3b

Fig. 3 *a-e. Arteriovenous malformation associated with an intradiploic angioma.* 18-year-old man. *a,* axial, T1W; *b,* axial, spin-echo proton density-weighted (PW); *c,* axial, spin-echo T2-weighted (T2W); *d,* axial, GRE T1W MR images; and *e,* axial, 3D-TOF MRA.

A left frontal, parenchymal arteriovenous malformation is seen in all the pulse sequences (curved arrows). Of particular note is a intradiploic angiomatous lesion (a small angioma or hemangioma) is associated with the condition, which is unremarkable on T1W (*a*), and PW (*b*) images, and is bright on the T2W image (arrows, *c*), and on the flow-sensitive GRE, T1W image (arrow, *d*). It is also seen on the 3D-TOF MRA (arrow, *e*). Note that the involved diploe is normal in thickness (compare with the contralateral diploe). Plain X-rays and CT scans were unremarkable for the intradiploic lesion. Diploic venous lakes may give a similar appearance on the T2W image, however, they are usually identified on plain X-rays and CT scans.

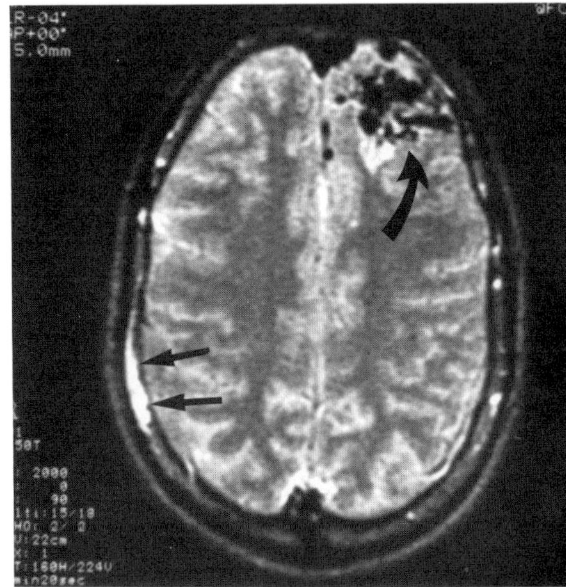

3c

3d

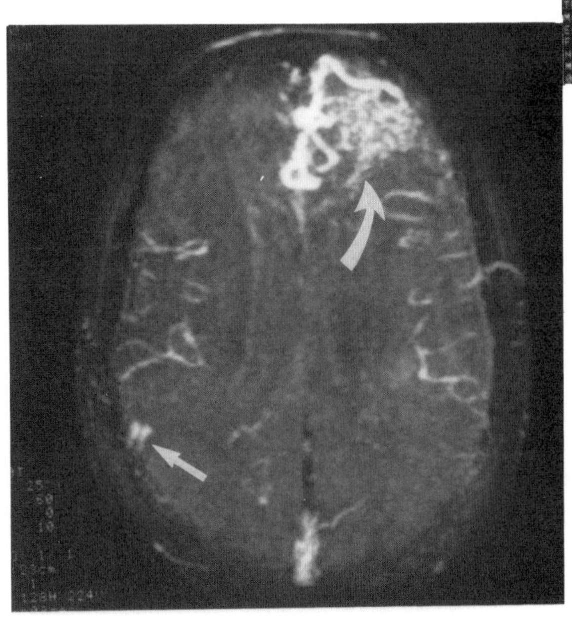

3e

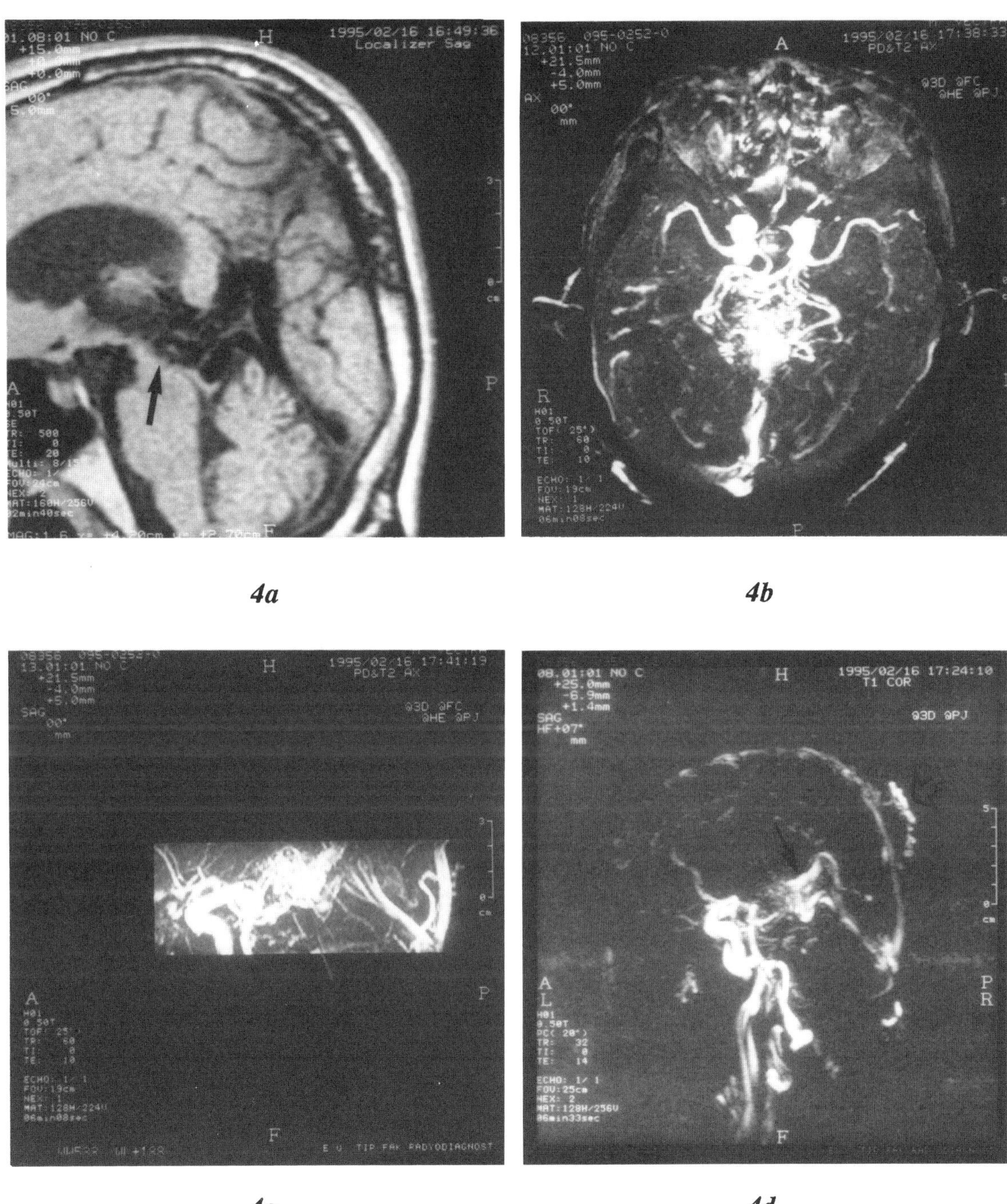

4a   4b

4c   4d

Fig. 4 *a-d. Arteriovenous malformation associated with a subcutaneous vascular malformation.* 10-year-old boy. *a,* sagittal T1W; *b,* axial 3D-TOF MRA; *c,* sagittal 3D-TOF MRA; and *d,* sagittal 3D-PC MRA. There is an arteriovenous malformation involving the midbrain (arrows, *a-d*), drained by a slightly enlarged vein of Galen, and an accessory venous structure. Sagittal 3D-PC MRA demonstrates an accompanying subcutaneous vascular malformation (open arrow, *d*).

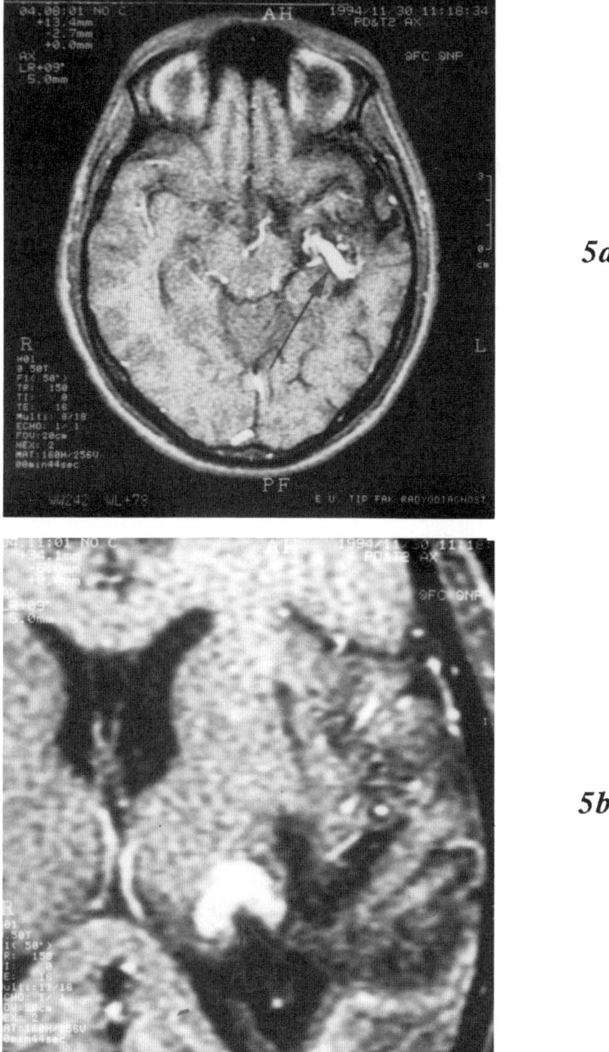

5a

5b

Fig. 5 *a-e. **Arteriovenous malformation associated with hemorrhage.*** Adult patient. *a,* axial GRE T1W; *b,* axial GRE T1W; *c,* axial T2W; *d,* axial 3D-TOF MRA; and *e,* axial 3D-PC MRA. An arteriovenous malformation in seen (arrows, *a,d,e*) supplied by the left middle cerebral artery. There is   subacute bleeding in the left thalamus giving high-signal both on the GRE T1W (*b*), and T2W (*c*) images representing presence of extracellular methemoglobin, a subacute phase blood product created after bleeding (open arrows, *b,c*). Blood products at different phases are also seen at the region of external capsule and claustrum (*b,c*). Note that the subacute phase blood product is seen on the 3D-TOF image (open arrow, *d*), a consequence of the Maximum Intensity Projection (MIP) reconstruction of 3D-TOF images, causing a limitation for the technique (hyperintense background). Similar T1-sensitivity creating a hyperintense background is also seen with fat and contrast medium on 3D-TOF MRA. Note that the arteriovenous malformation is better seen on the 3D-PC MRA (*e*), a technique with good background suppression.

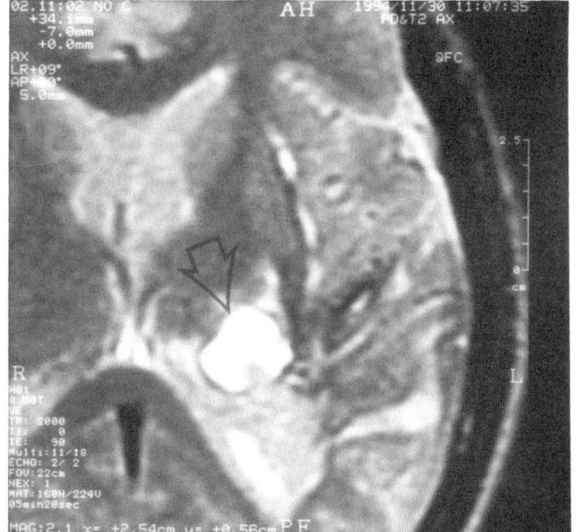

5c

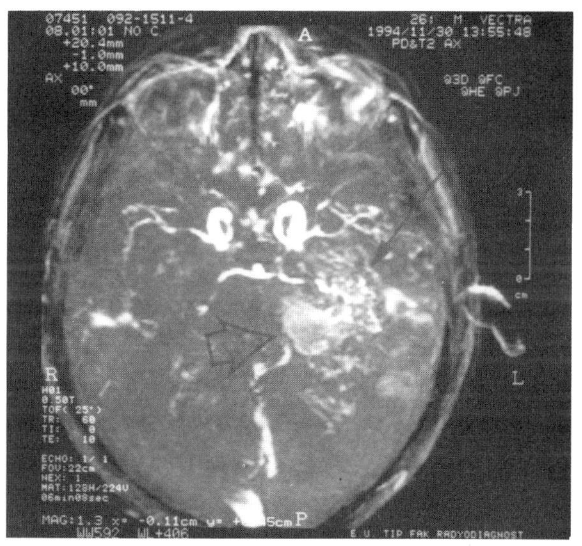

5d

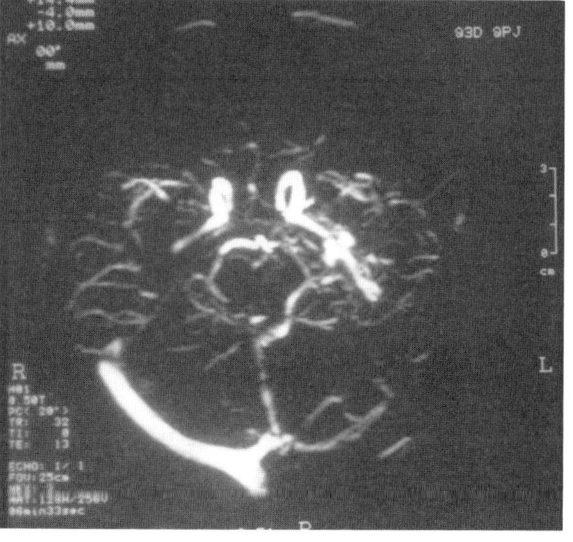

5e

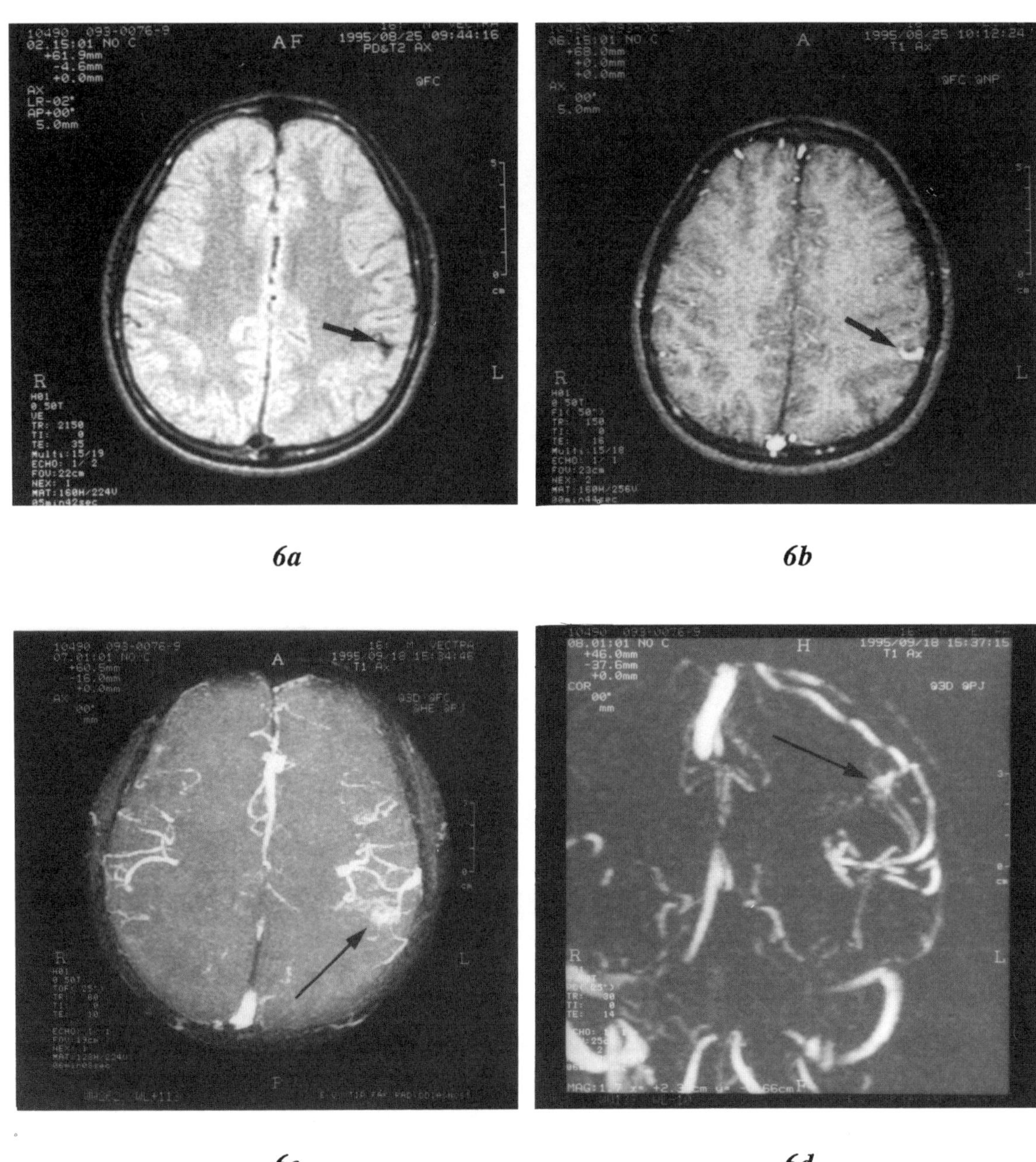

6a   *6b*

6c   *6d*

Fig. 6 *a-d. Small arteriovenous malformation.* 16-year-old boy. *a,* axial PDW; *b,* axial GRE T1W; *c,* axial 3D-TOF MRA; and *d,* coronal 3D-PC MRA. There is a small parenchymal focus in the left parietal region, which is hypointense on the PDW image, and hyperintense on the GRE T1W image (arrows, *a,b*). MR angiography clearly identifies this focus as a small arteriovenous malformation (arrows *c,d*).

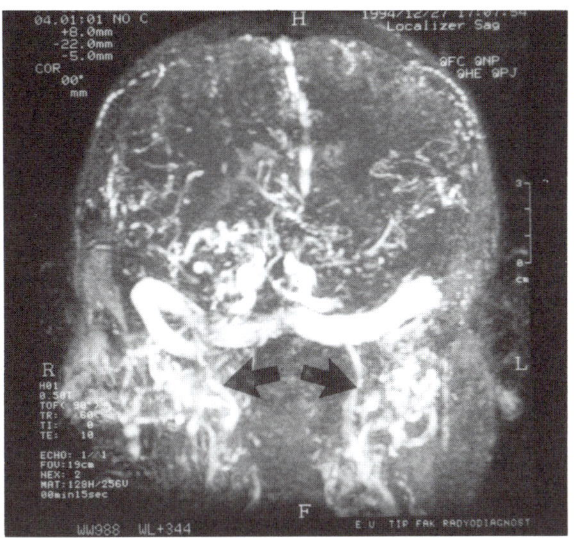

7a

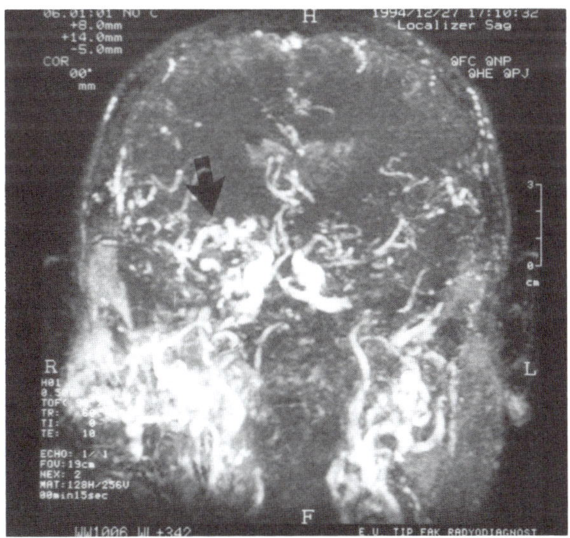

7b

Fig. 7 *a, b. Dural arteriovenous malformation.* Adult patient. *a,* and *b,* coronal 2-dimensional time-of-flight MR angiography (2D-TOF MRA) images. A network of multiple dilated vessels representing an extensive dural arteriovenous malformation involving the posterior cranial fossa, and the supratentorial region is well demonstrated (arrows).

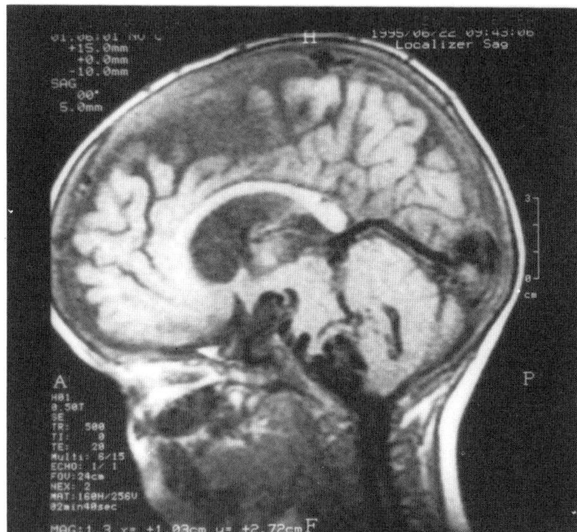

8a

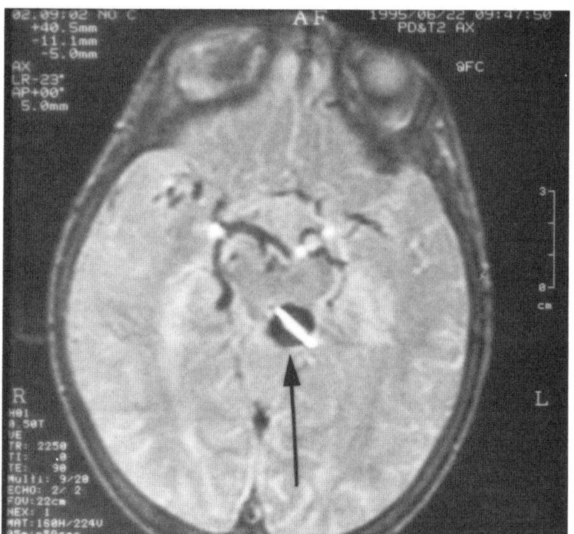

8b

Fig. 8 *a-e. Aneurysm associated with mixed arteriovenous malformation.* 2-year-old boy. *a,* sagittal T1W; *b,* axial T2W; *c,* GRE T1W; *d,* sagittal 3D-PC MRA; and *e,* axial 3D-PC MRA. T1W image shows multiple dilated vessels in the posterior fossa located within the parenchymal structures and peripherally *(a).* There is an aneurysm originating from the left posterior cerebral artery (arrows, *b-d*), and a network of vessels representing an extensive mixed arteriovenous malformation (open arrows, *d,e*).

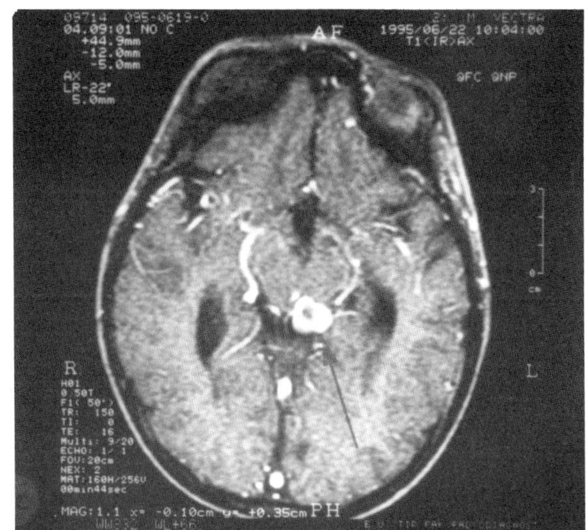

8c

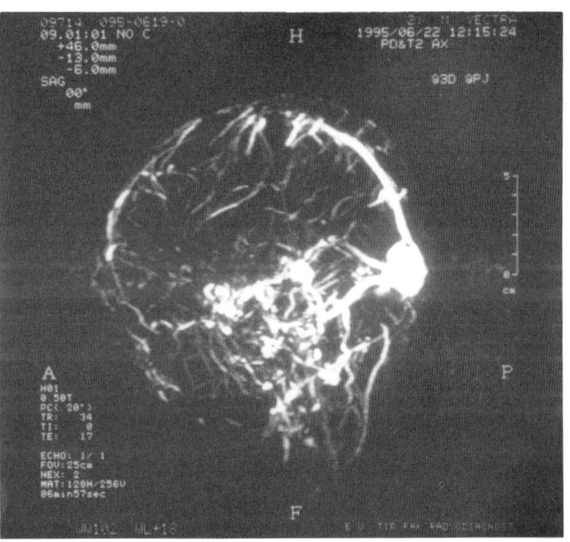

8d

8e

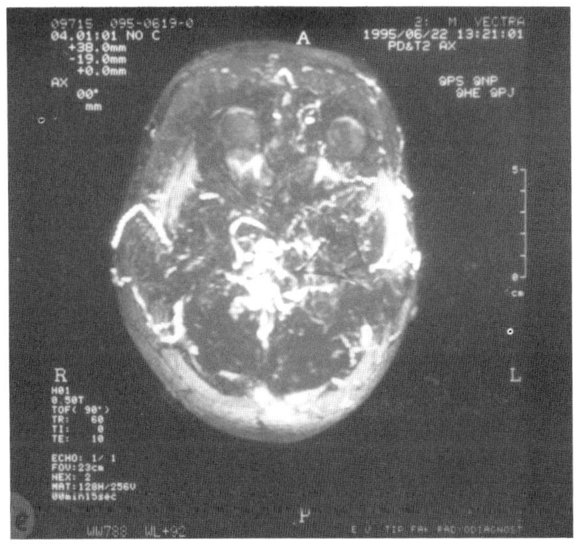

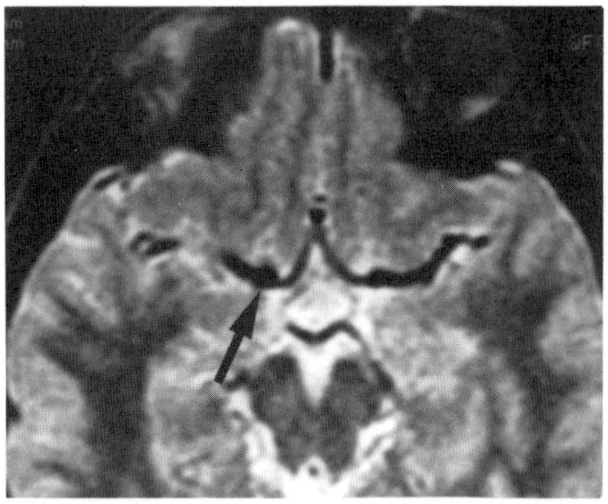

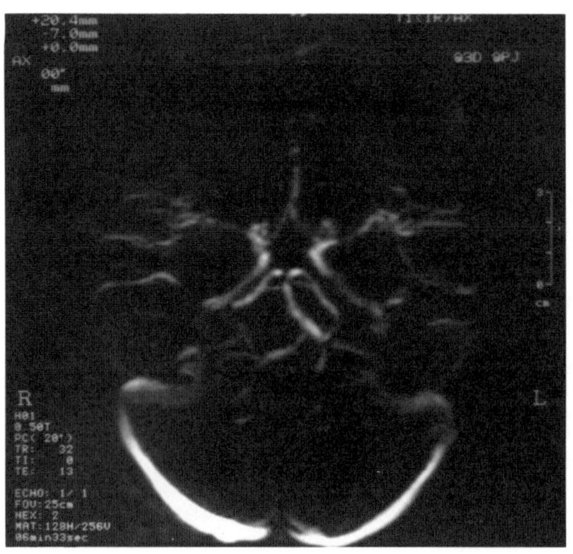

9a

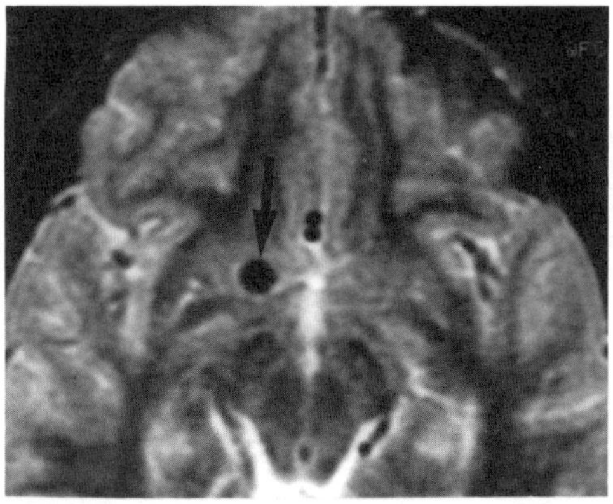

9b

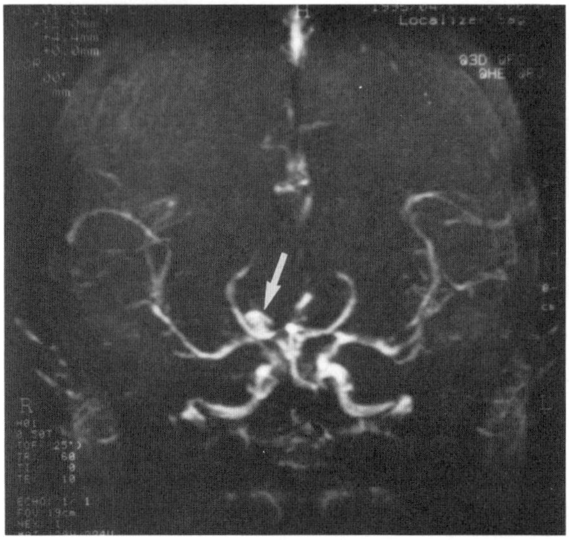

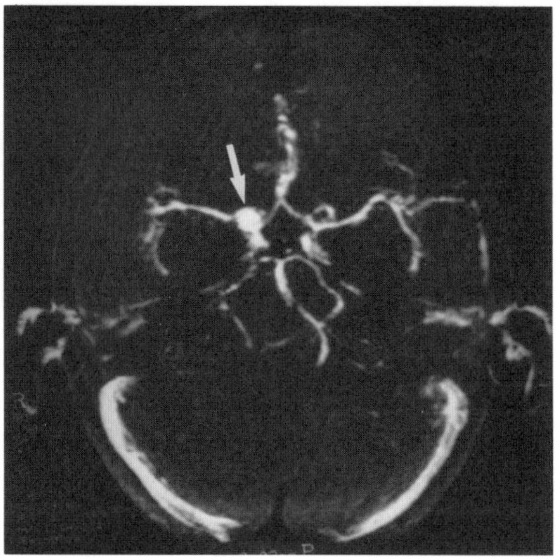

9c

9d

9e

Fig. 9 *a-e*. *Aneurysm (a pitfall of 3D-PC MRA)*. 9-year-old girl. *a,* axial, T2W; *b,* axial, T2W; *c,* coronal, 3D-TOF MRA; *d,* axial, 3D-TOF MRA; and *e,* axial, 3D-PC MRA.

T2W images show an aneurysm of 8mm diameter at the right internal carotid bifurcation (arrows, *a,b*). 3D-TOF MRA's readily demonstrate the lesion in axial (*c*) and coronal (*d*) projections (arrows). 3D-PC MRA, however, fails to demonstrate the lesion *(e)*. Recent reports emphasized such a pitfall of 3D-PC MRA especially in aneurysms of smaller sizes.

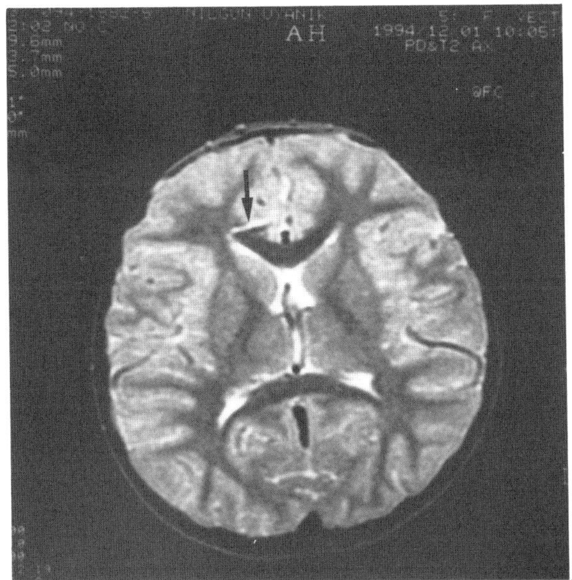

10a

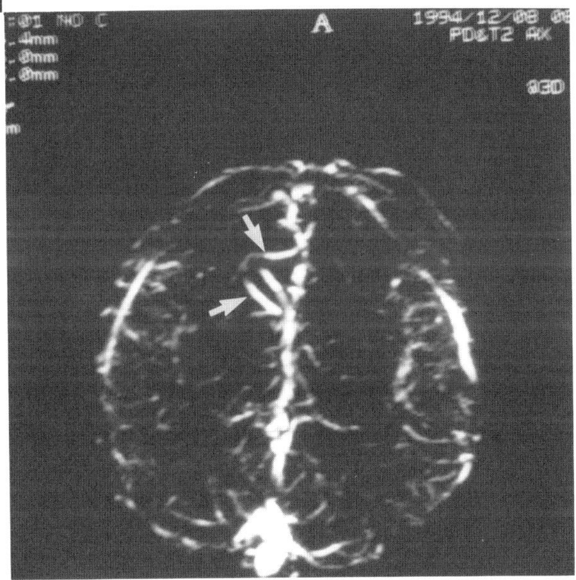

10b

Fig. 10 *a, b. Venous malformation.* 5-year-old girl. *a,* axial, T2W; and *b,* axial, 3D-PC MRA (velocity=6cm/sec).

A venous malformation is seen both on the T2W image (arrow, *a*), and 3D-PC MRA (velocity=6cm/sec, an axial slab centered to the centrum semiovale) (arrow, *b*). Although, a venous malformation can readily be detected on spin-echo or gradient recalled-echo images, their demonstration by MR angiography may be problematic. They may be seen on a 2-dimensional time-of-flight MR angiography (2D-TOF MRA), but a 3D-TOF MRA is usually negative. A 3D-PC MRA with a low flow velocity (i.e. 6cm/sec) is usually required for their demonstration. Venous malformations may be considered as extreme variations of normal.

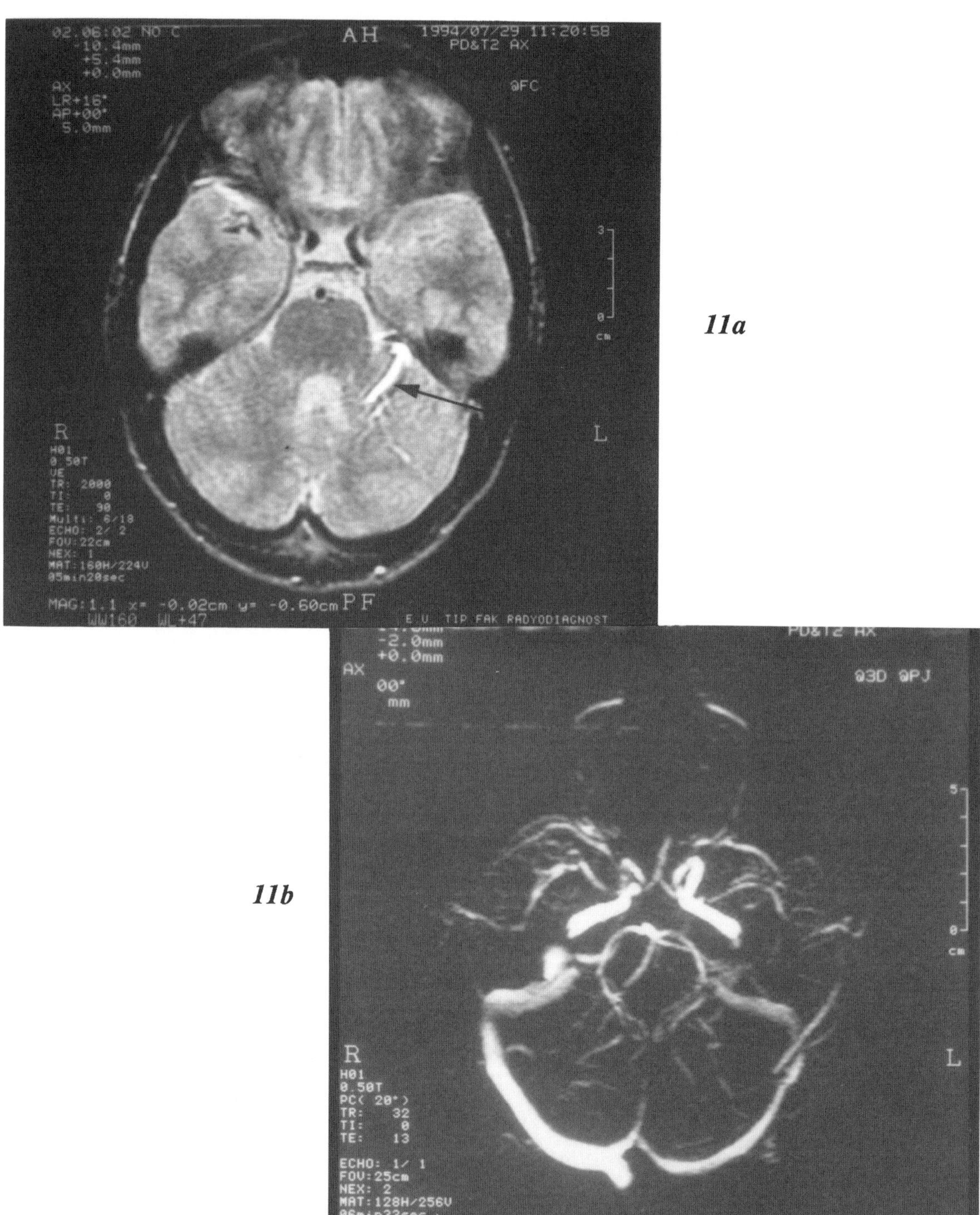

Fig. 11 *a, b. Venous malformation (a pitfall of 3D-PC MRA).* Adult patient. *a,* axial T2W; and *b,* axial 3D-PC MRA (velocity = 21 cm/sec). T2W image shows a venous malformation in the left cerebellar hemisphere with classical features; a spoke-wheel pattern caused by multiple converging venules, drained by a large venous structure (arrow). 3D-PC MRA obtained utilizing a relatively high velocity (21 cm/sec) fails to demonstrate the venous malformation (see Fig.10).

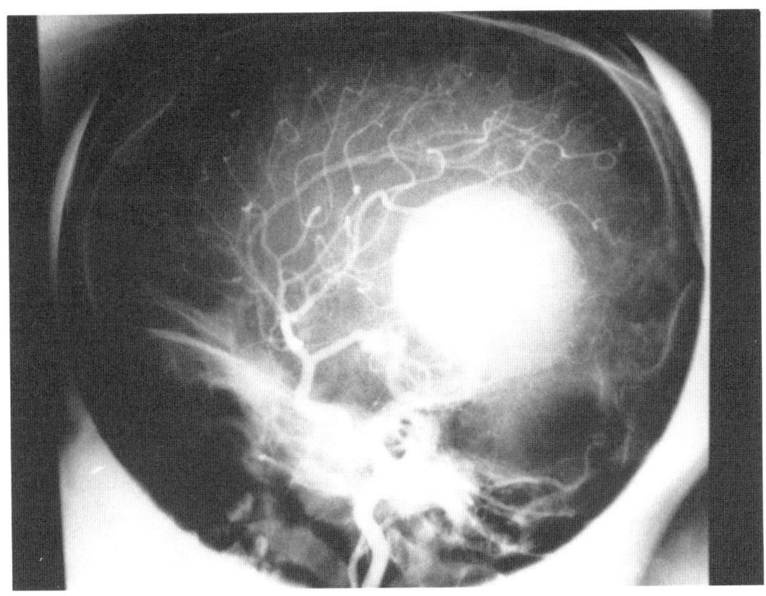

12a

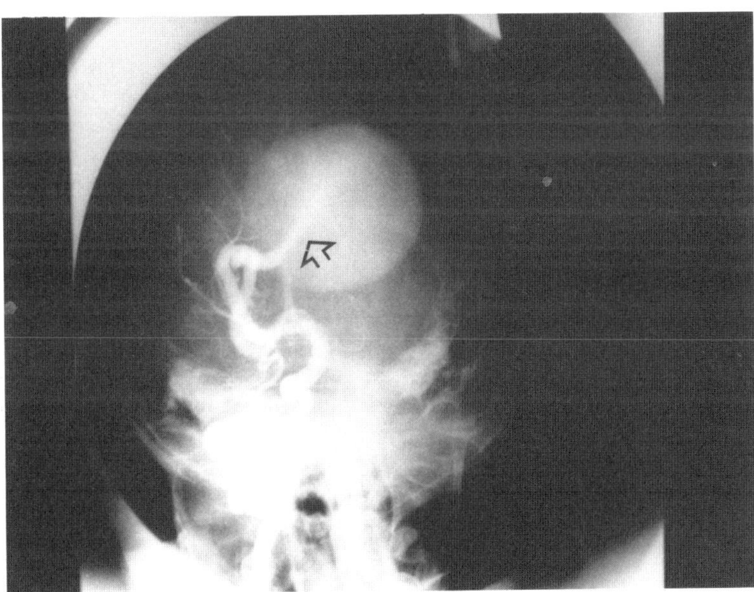

12b

Fig.12 *a-f. Vein of Galen malformation.* 6-year-old girl. *a,b,* and *c,* conventional angiograms; and *d,* sagittal 3D-PC MRA (velocity = 21 cm/sec); *e,* axial, 3D-PC MRA (velocity = 21 cm/sec); and *f,* coronal, 3D-TOF MRA.

Conventional angiograms show a large vein of Galen malformation. Note a "jet" of flow from the posterior cerebral artery into the malformation (arrow, *b*). There is venous constraint in the straight sinus (small arrow) and transverse sinus (long arrow) (*c*). The 3D-PC MRA,

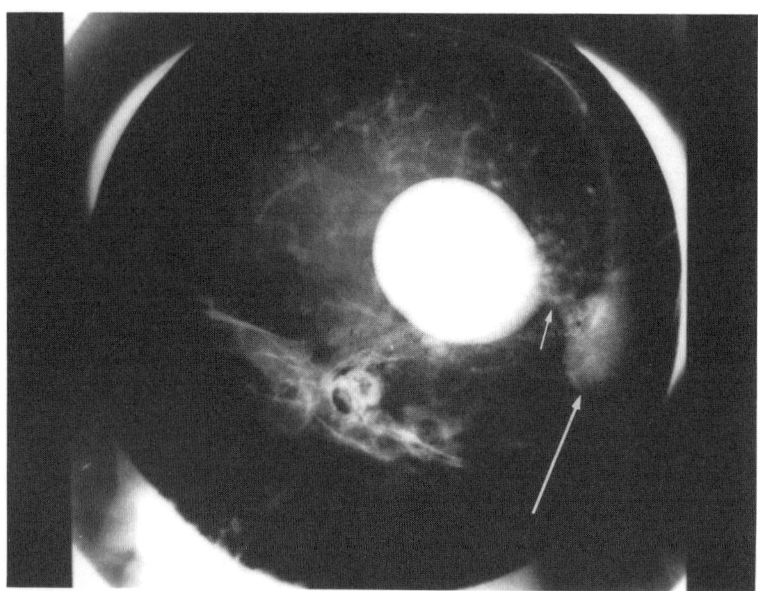

12c

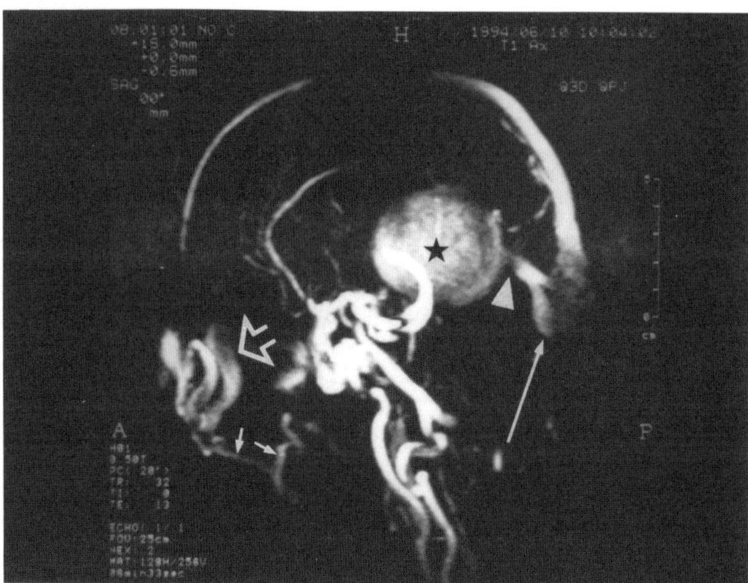

12d

and the 3D-TOF MRA show comparable changes; the enlarged vein of Galen (stars, *d,e,f*), a direct arteriovenous fistula (curved arrow, *e*), the venous constraint in the straight sinus (arrowhead, *d* ; arrows, *e*), and transverse sinus (long arrow, *d*). Main venous outflow is through the enlarged right superior opthalmic vein (open arrows *d,e*), and facial veins (small arrows, *d*). From embryologic point of view, such a malformation related with the vein of Galen actually represents an "aneurysm of the persistent, primitive prosencephalic vein of Markowski" (from reference 33).

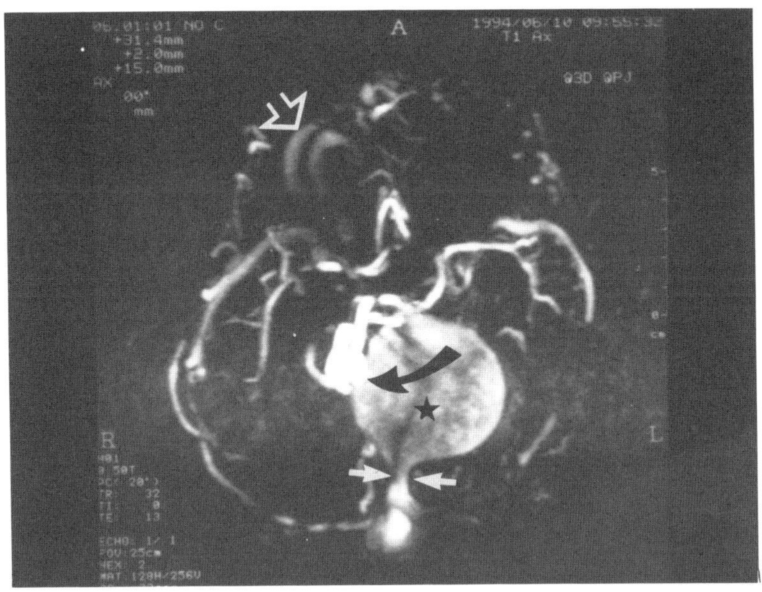

12e

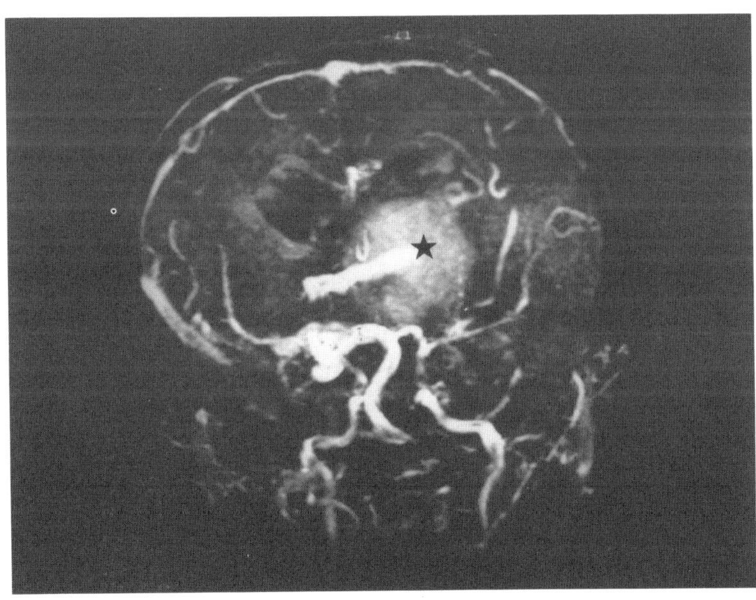

12f

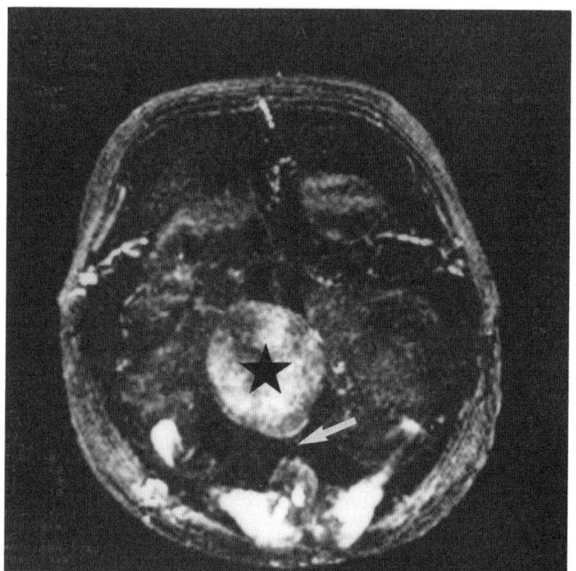

13a

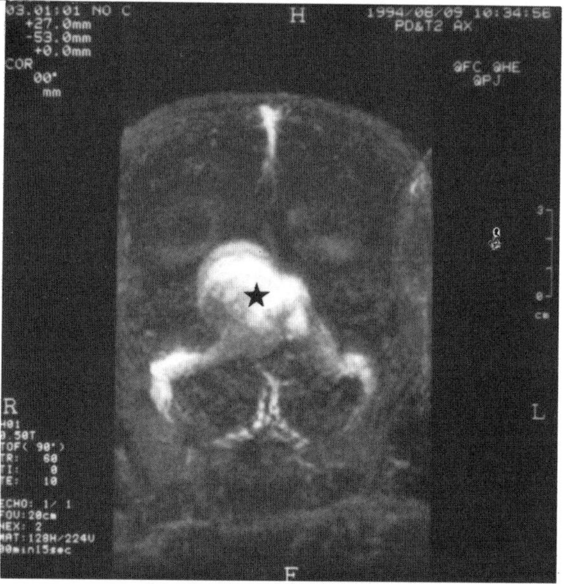

13b

Fig. 13 *a,b*. *Vein of Galen malformation*. 5-month-old boy. *a,* axial 2-dimensional time-of-flight MR angiography (2D-TOF MRA); *b,* coronal 2D-TOF MRA.

The dilated vein of Galen is seen (stars). Note restriction to venous outflow in the straight sinus (arrow, *a*) (from reference 33).

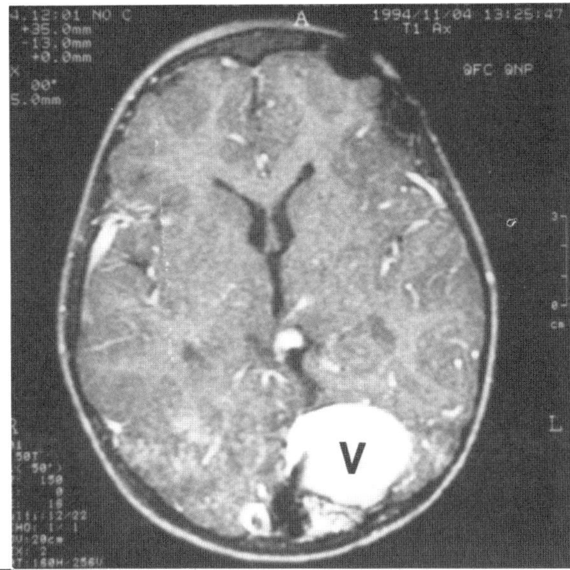

14a

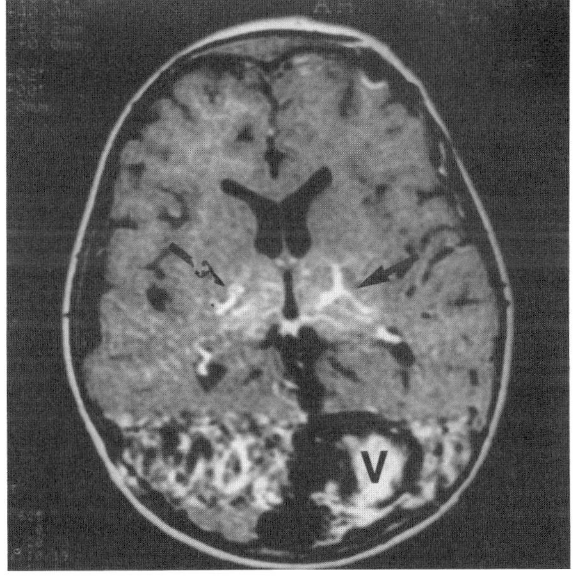

14b

**Fig.14 a-d . *Varix of the torcula and dural sinuses associated with mixed arterio-venous malformations.* 4.5-year-old boy. *a,* axial, GRE T1W; *b,* axial, T1W (after administration of contrast medium); *c,* coronal, 2D-TOF MRA; and *d,* axial, 3D-TOF MRA.

A large torcular varix (V) is seen on the GRE, T1W (*a*) T1W (after administration of contrast medium) (*b*), and 2D-TOF MRA (*c*). It loses signal on the 3D-TOF MRA (*d*) due to turbulent flow. Superior sagittal, right transverse and sigmoid sinuses show apparent ectasia (*c,d*). Note multiple, enlarged medullary veins at the region of the thalami (arrows, *b*) , and in the hemispheres (arrows, *c*). The left posterior cerebral artery, and several branches off the middle cerebral arteries reach to the superficial veins and directly communicate with a network of abnormal vessels (arrows, *d*).

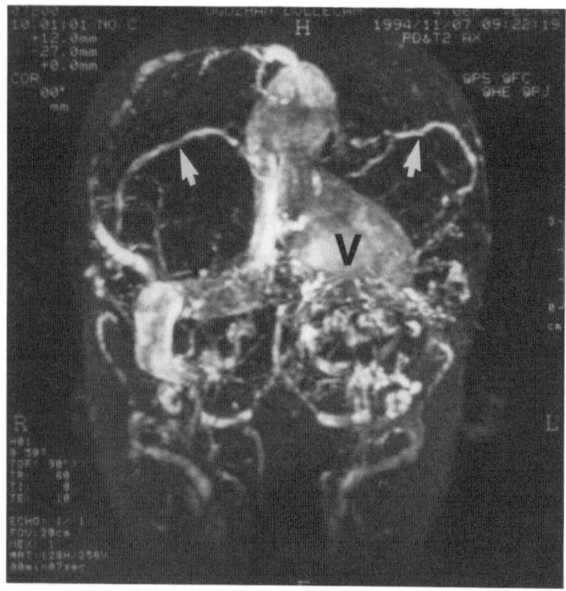

14c

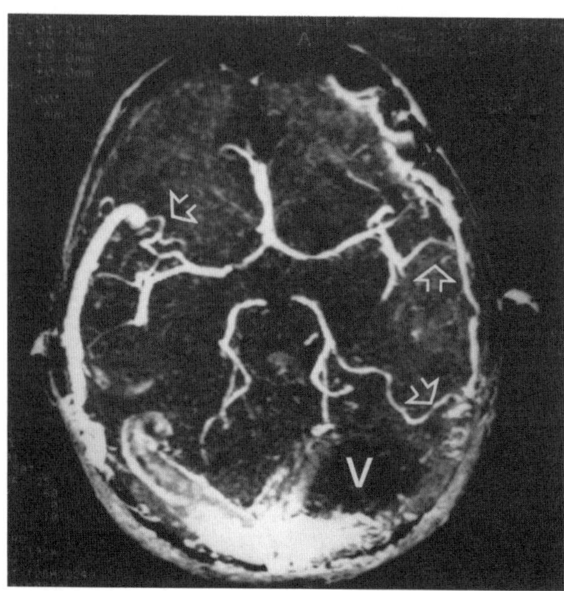

14d

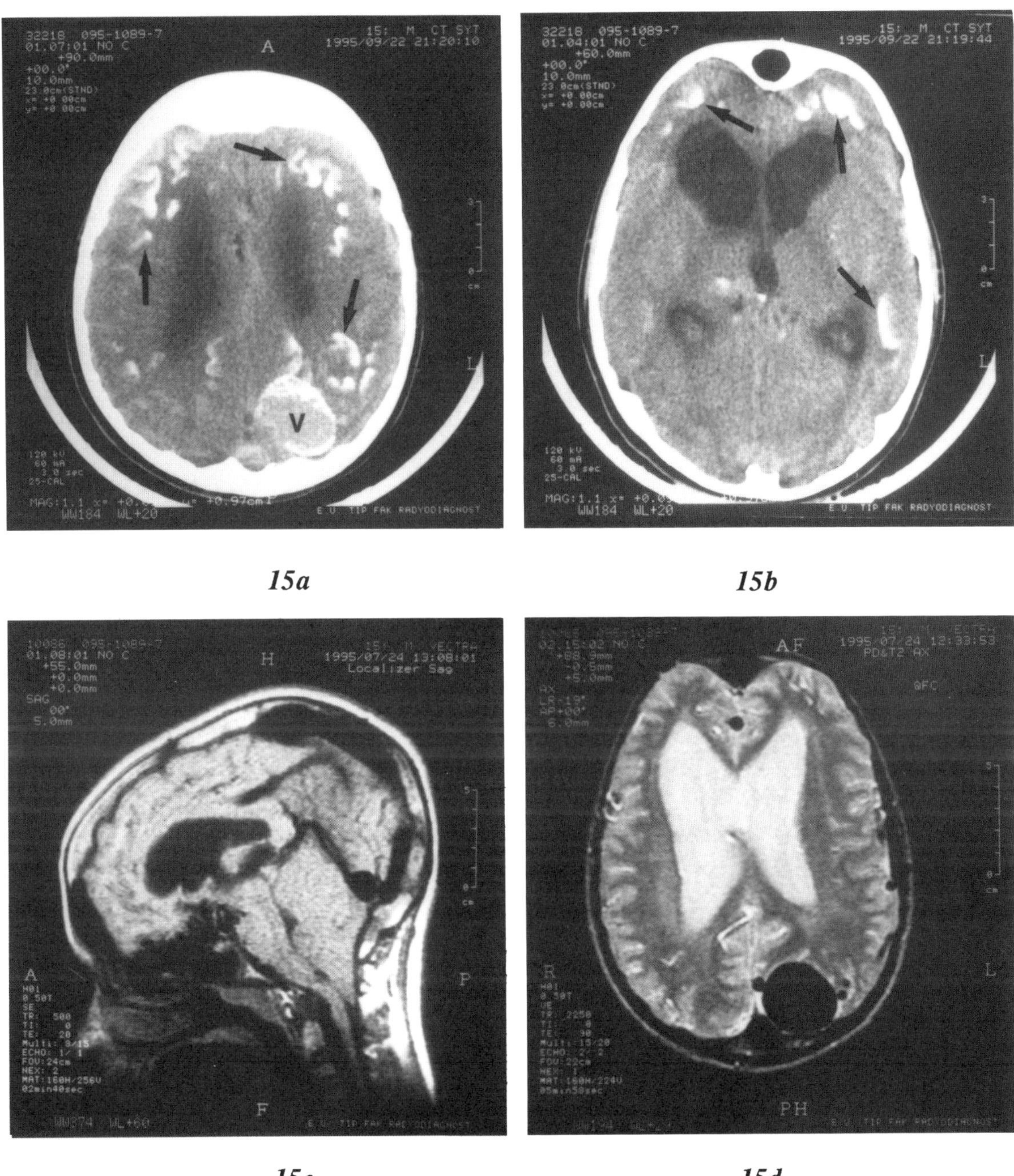

15a   15b

15c   15d

Fig.15 *a-j*. *Varix of the dural sinus, arteriovenous malformation, mineralizing microangiopathy, and an abnormal cerebellum.* 15-year-old boy. *a* and *b,* CT scans; *c,* sagittal T1W; *d,* axial T2W; *e,* axial GRE T1W; *f,* axial 3D-TOF MRA; *g,* coronal 2D-TOF MRA; *h,* sagittal 3D-PC MRA; and *i* and *j,* conventional angiograms. CT scans show extensive gyriform calcifications located at the corticomedullary junction (arrows, *a,b*). These calcifications have an identical pattern to the so-called mineralizing microangiopathy

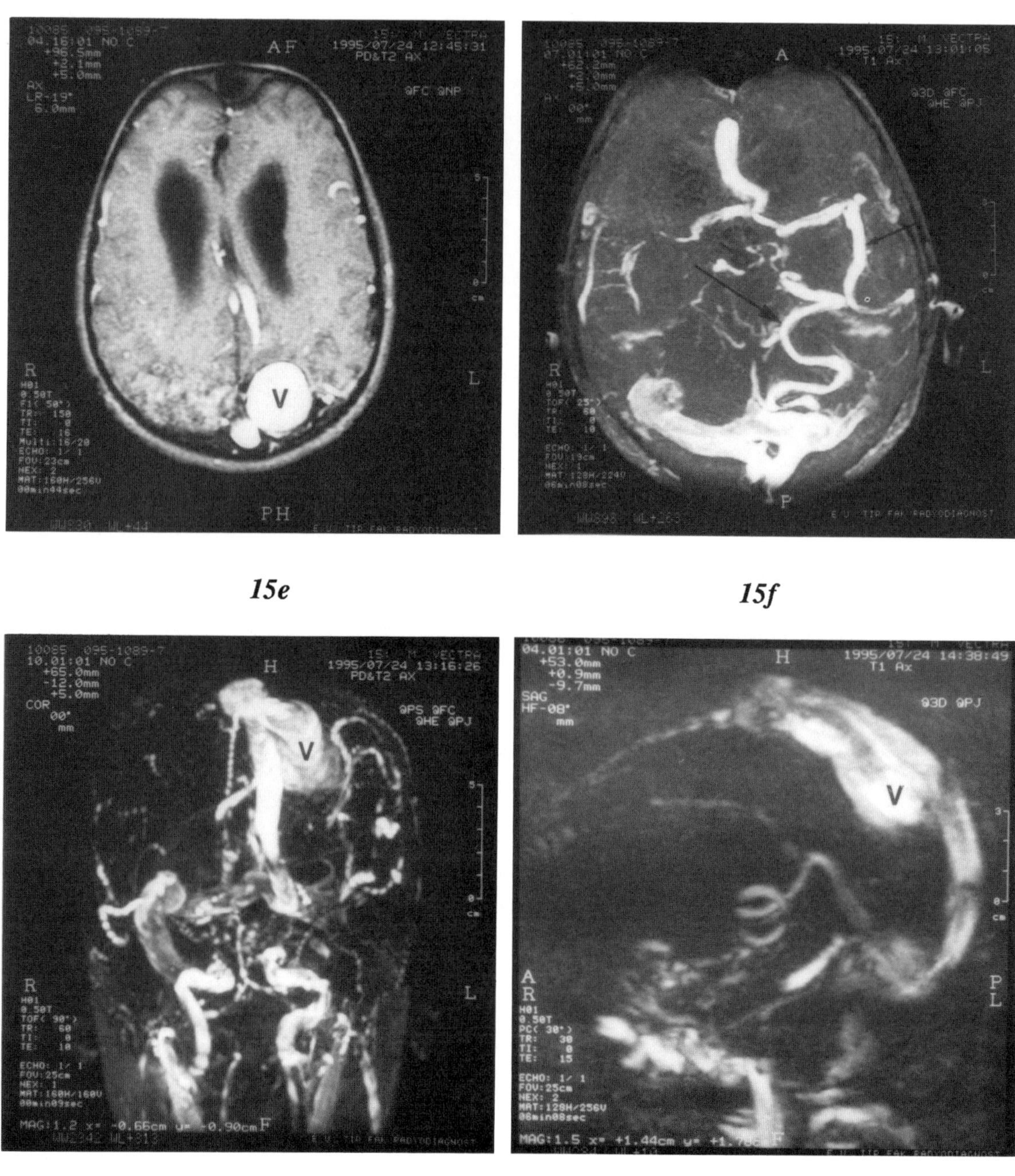

15e

15f

15g

15h

which is known to be associated with vasculopathy and dystrophic calcification at the corticomedullary junction, and the basal ganglia, and usually develops after combined chemotherapy and radiation treatment of the central nervous system tumors in childhood. The calcifications in this 15-year-old patient may have resulted from a long-standing vasculopathy and dystrophic calcification. There is a calcified varix (V) connected with the superior sagittal sinus (*a*). Conventional angiography demonstrates a nidus of parenchymal

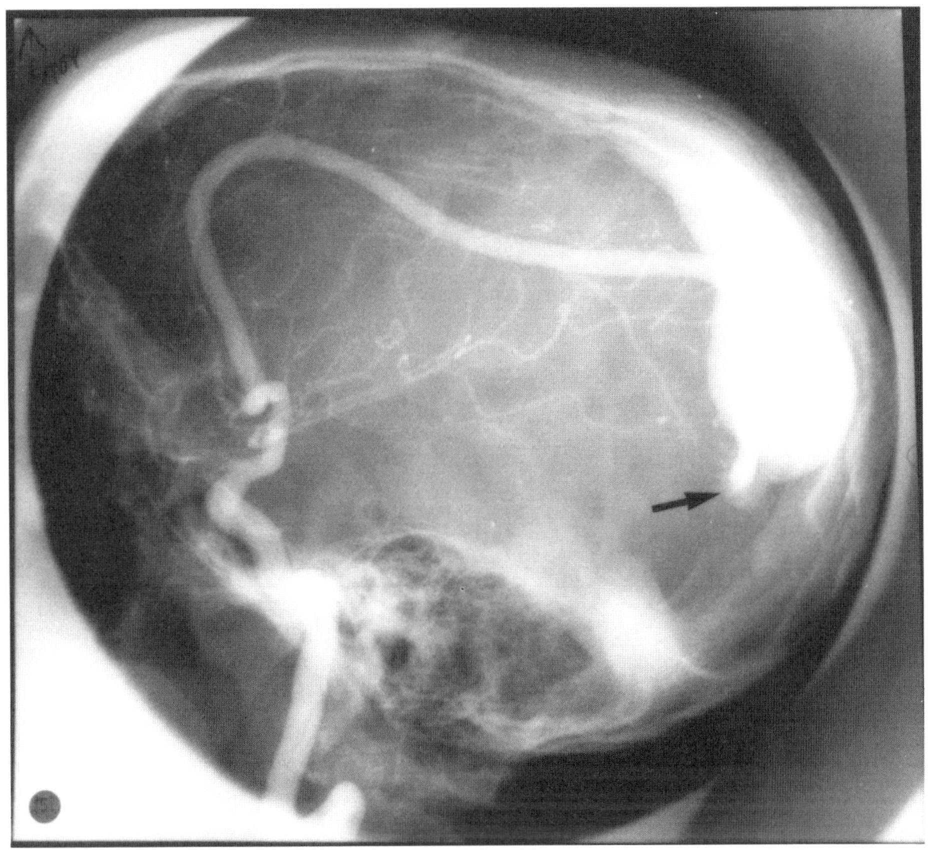

15i

arteriovenous malformation (arrows, *i, j*), supplied by the anterior and middle cerebral arteries, which drains to the dural varix and to the dilated superior sagittal sinus. 3D-TOF MRA shows the dilated middle cerebral (short arrow), and posterior cerebral (long arrow) arteries also supplying the arteriovenous malformation (*f*). T2W and GRE T1W images show the varix (V), as well as the 2D-TOF MRA, and 3D-PC MRA *(g,h)*. Note that the varix appears to have a narrow connection to the superior sagittal sinus *(d,e)*. The cerebellum is abnormal; there is herniation of the tonsillas into the cervical canal, and the superior vermis shows towering (it is high) such as that seen in Chiari II malformation (*c*). However, radiography, physical examination and patient history excluded a spinal defect, which is seen in almost all the patients with Chiari II malformation.

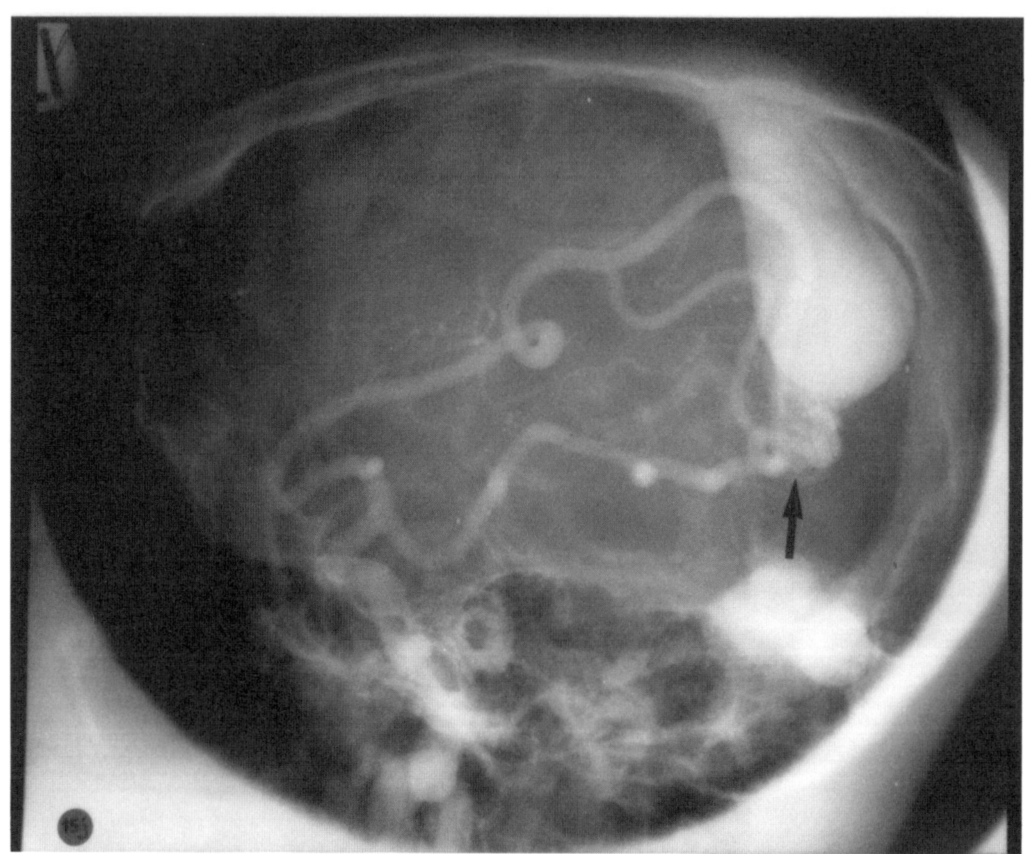

15j

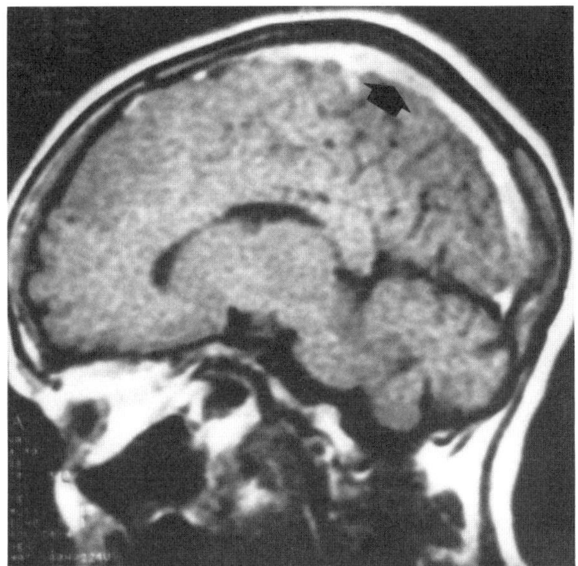

16a

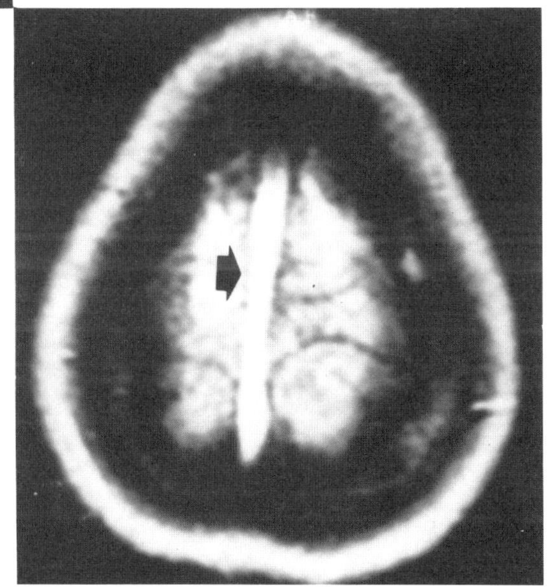

16b

Fig. 16 *a-f. Dural sinus thrombosis.* Adult patient. *a,* sagittal, T1W; *b,* axial, T2W; *c,* axial, PW; *d,* axial, T2W; *e,* coronal, 3D-PC MRA (velocity = 21cm/sec); and *f,* axial, 3D-PC MRA (velocity = 21cm/sec).

High signal is evident in the superior sagittal sinus and right sigmoid sinus on T1W, PW, and T2W images suggesting presence of a subacute thrombus (extracellular methemoglobin) (arrows, *a, b, c*). There are scattered venous infarcts (stars, *d*). 3D-PC MRA's reveal that the superior sagittal, right transverse and sigmoid sinuses, and the right jugular vein are not seen due to thrombosis.

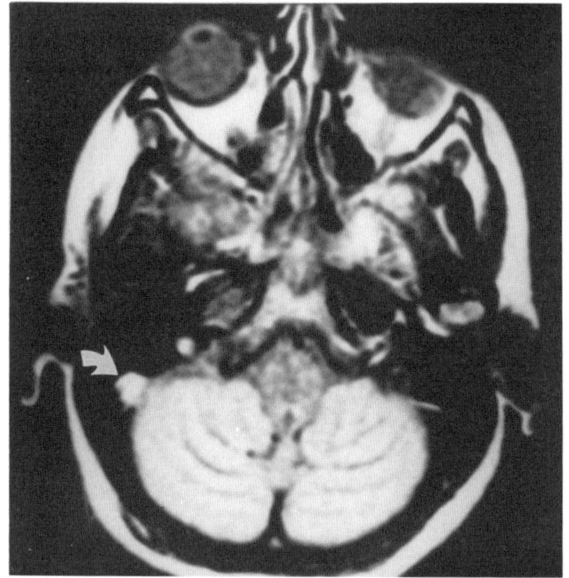

16c

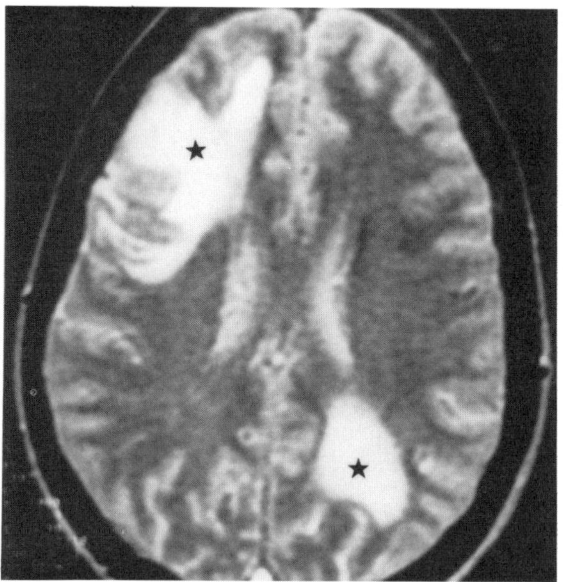

16d

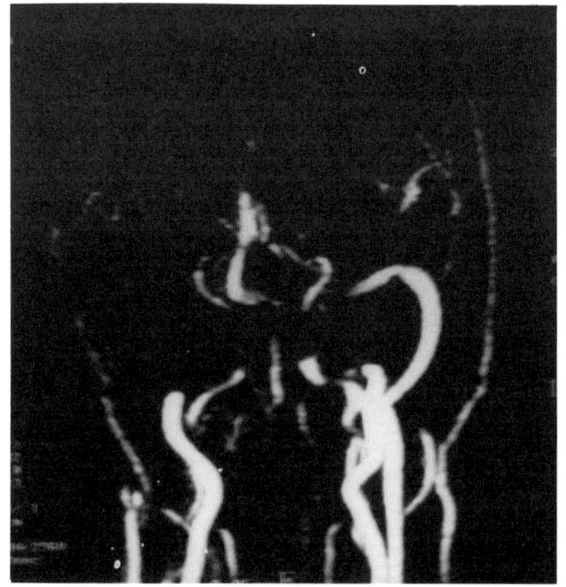

16e

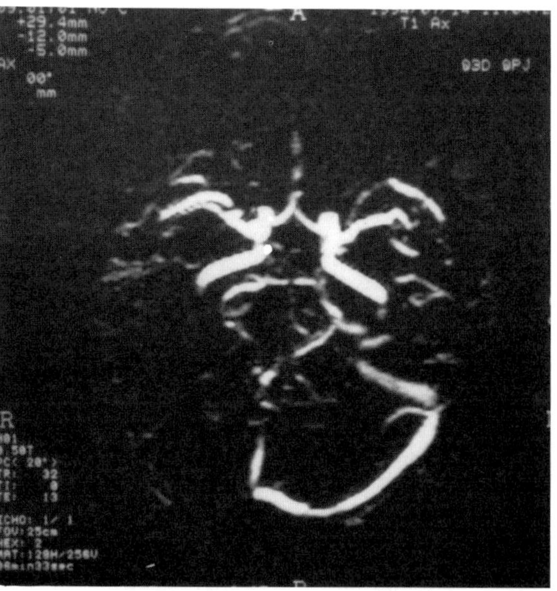

16f

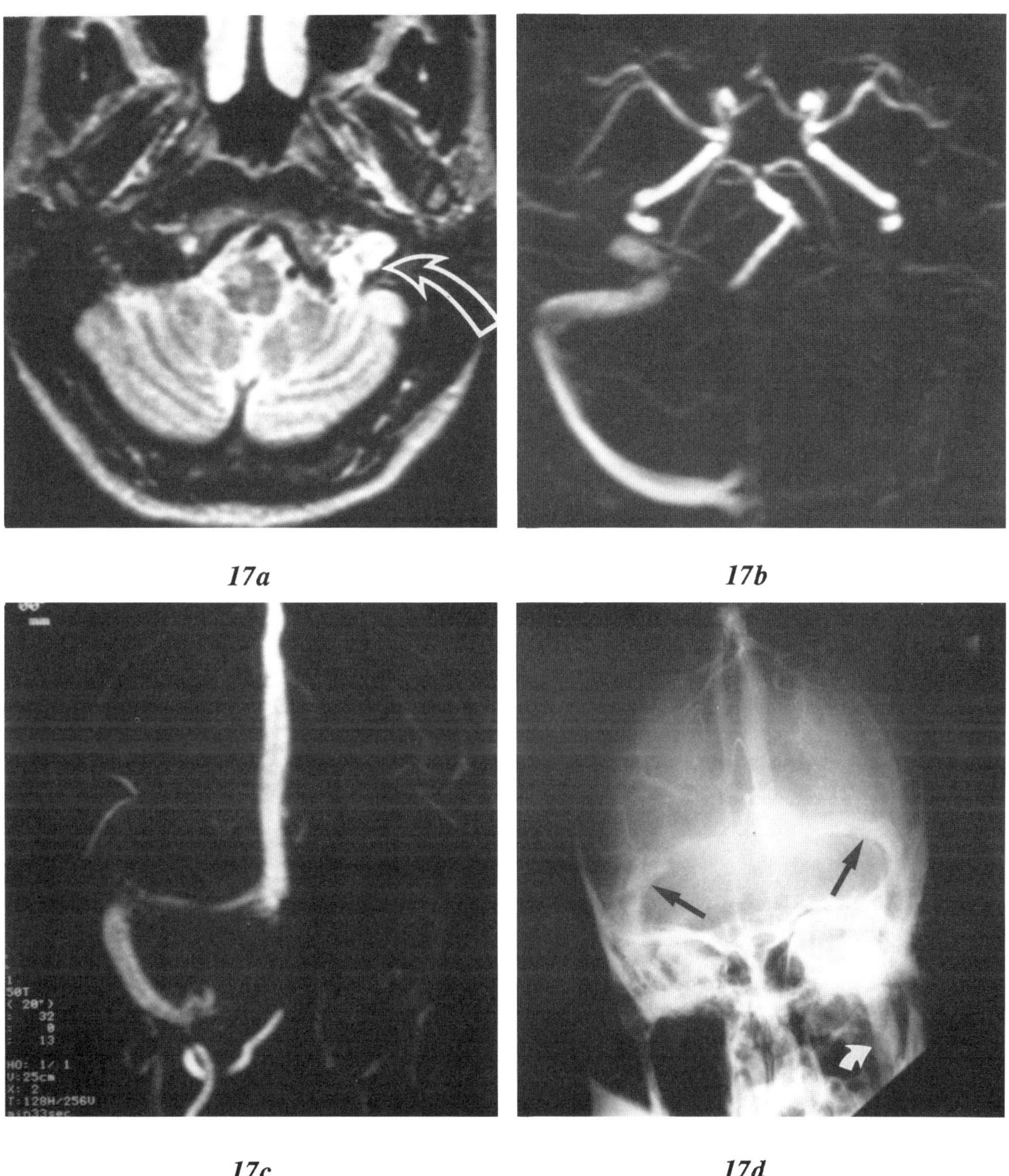

17a   *17b*

17c   *17d*

Fig.17 *a-f.   Normal jugular vein with slow flow (A pitfall of 3D-PC MRA causing a false diagnosis of venous thrombosis).*   Adult patient. *a,* axial, T2W; *b,* axial, 3D-PC MRA (velocity = 20cm/sec); *c,* coronal 3D-PC MRA (velocity = 20cm/sec); *d,* conventional angiography; *e,* axial, 3D-PC MRA (velocity = 7cm/sec); *f,* axial, 2D-TOF MRA.

T2W image shows high signal in the left sigmoid sinus and jugular vein (arrow, *a*), suggesting a thrombotic event. 3D-PC MRA's with a velocity of 20cm/sec shows nonvisualization of the left transverse and sigmoid sinuses, and the jugular vein. These are

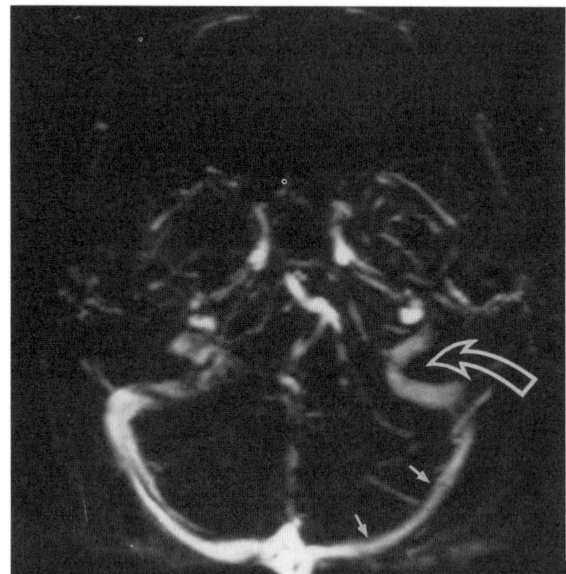

17e

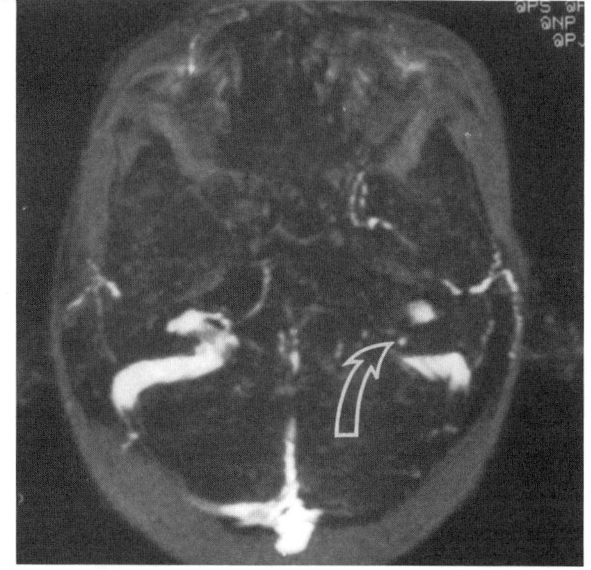

17f

normal on the right side *(b,c)*. Conventional angiography reveals that the sagittal, and both transverse and sigmoid sinuses are normal (straight arrows, *d*), as well as the left jugular vein (curved arrow, *d*). A repeat 3D-PC MRA with a velocity of 7cm/sec, reveals that the left transverse sinus (small arrows, *e*), and the sigmoid sinus, and the jugular vein (curved arrow, *e*) are all patent.

  2D-TOF MRA verifies that these are patent (arrow, *f*).

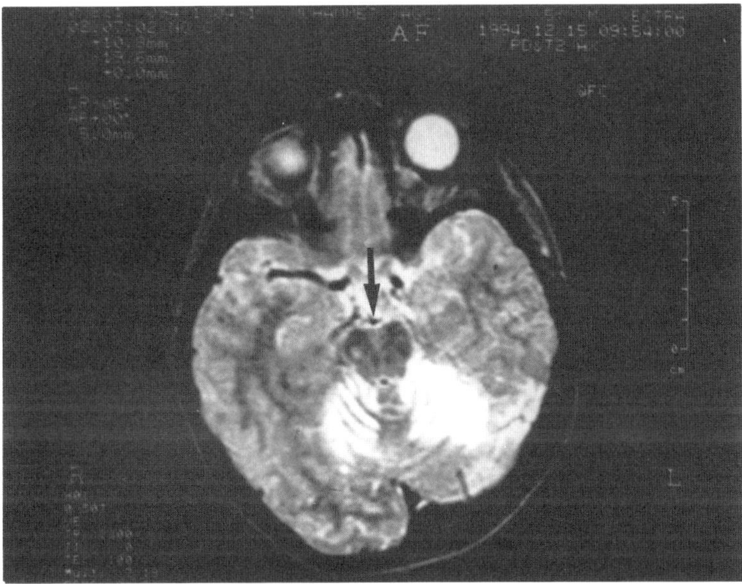

18a

Fig.18 *a-c. Traumatic vertebrobasilar dissection.* 5-year-old boy. *a,* axial, T2W; *b,* coronal, 3D-PC MRA (velocity = 21cm/sec); and *c,* follow-up axial, T2W image 3 months later.

T2W image shows hyperintensities in the cerebellum (at the territory of superior cerebellar arteries), in the pons, and in the left occipital region.

The basilar artery is narrow (arrow, *a*). 3D-PC MRA shows very poor visualization of the left vertebral artery (open arrow). The right vertebral artery is normal (small arrows), however, diminished luminal diameter of the basilar artery is noted, which reflects upward extension of the dissection in the left vertebral artery (*b*). T2W image obtained after three months shows the left vertebral artery with a patent lumen (arrow, *c*).

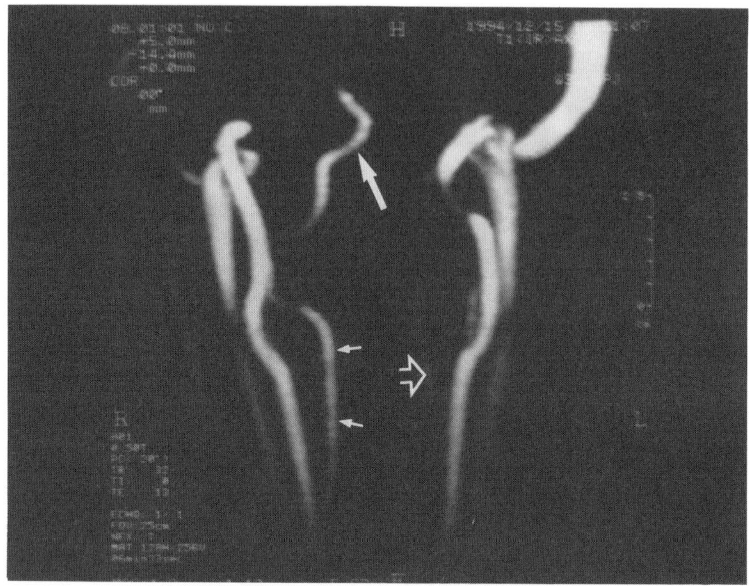

18b

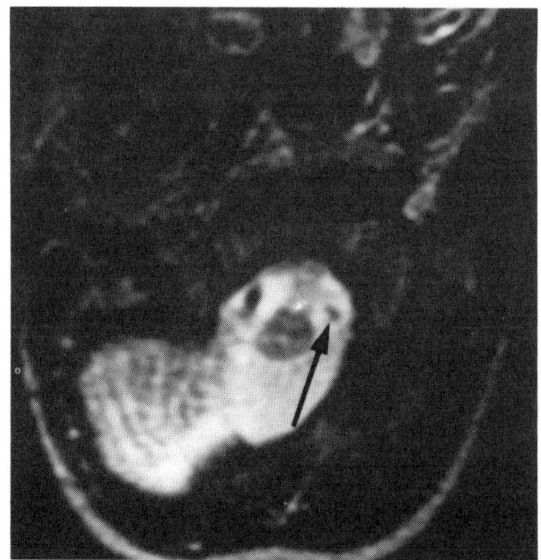

18c

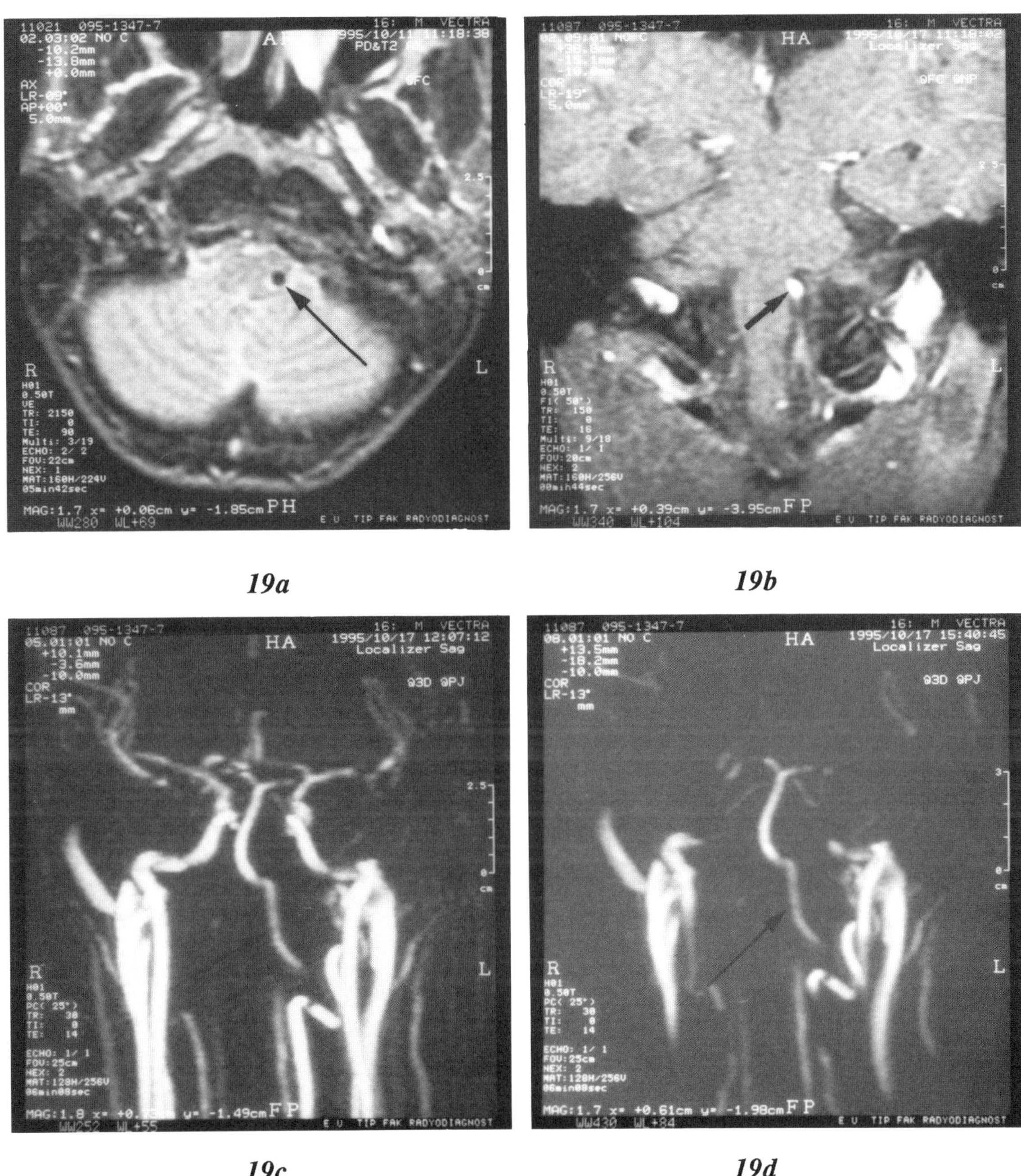

Fig.19 *a-d. Absence of the vertebral artery.* 16-year-old boy. *a,* axial T2W; *b,* coronal GRE T1W, *c* and *d,* coronal 3D-PC MRA (MIP reconstructions of 3D-PC MRA at two different planes). T2W image shows the flow-void of only the left vertebral artery (arrow, *a*), Coronal, GRE T1W image shows the bright signal of the left vertebral artery (arrow, *b*), however, the right vertebral artery is not seen. Coronal, 3D-PC MRA shows the normal left vertebral artery (arrows, *c,d*) The right vertebral artery is absent. Absence of the right vertebral artery was confirmed by conventional angiography.

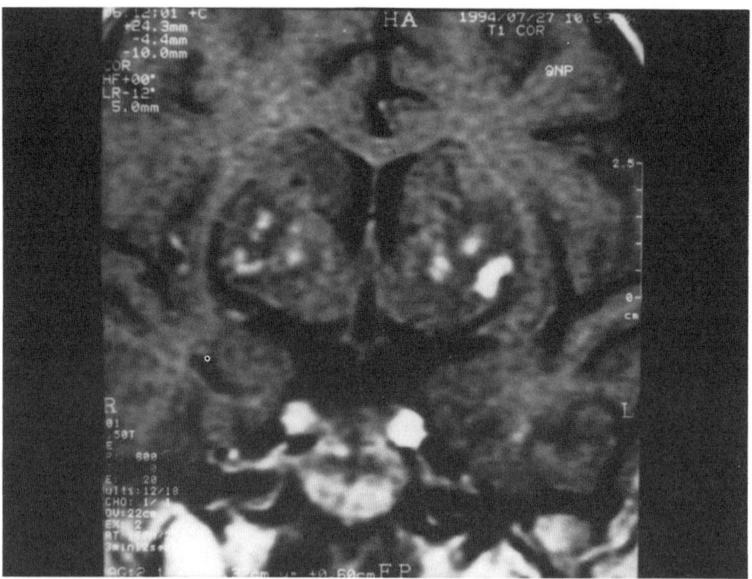

20a

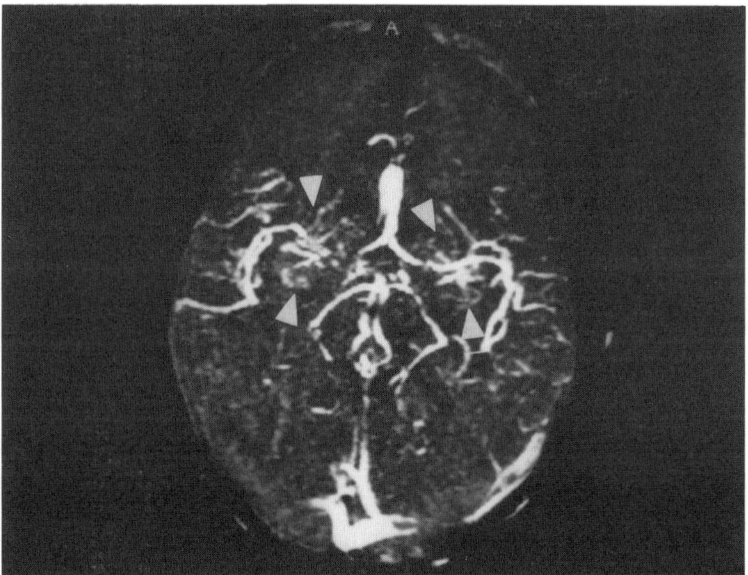

20b

Fig. 20 *a-d. Intracranial vasculitis.* 8-year-old girl. *a,* coronal, T1W (after administration of contrast medium); *b,* axial, 3D-TOF MRA; *c,* conventional angiography; and *d,* follow-up axial, T1W (after administration of contrast medium) 50 days later.

T1W image after administration of contrast medium shows multiple enhancing foci in the lentiform nuclei (*a*). 3D-TOF MRA shows an excessive number of small perforating arteries (arrowheads, *b*). Conventional angiography reveals prominent perforating vessels which show focal narrowings and dilatations, suggesting vasculitis (arrows, *c*). Note that the

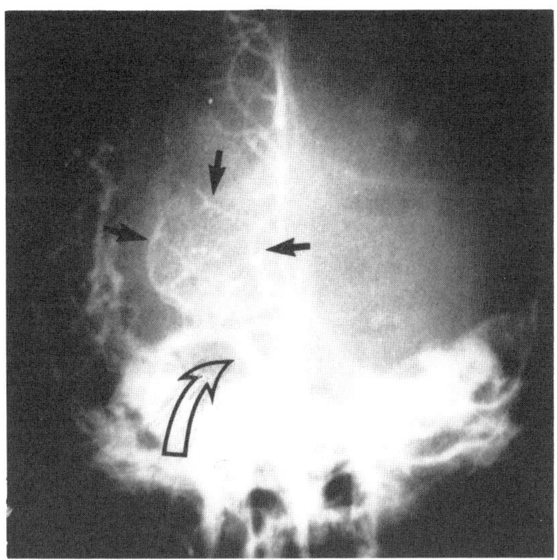

20c

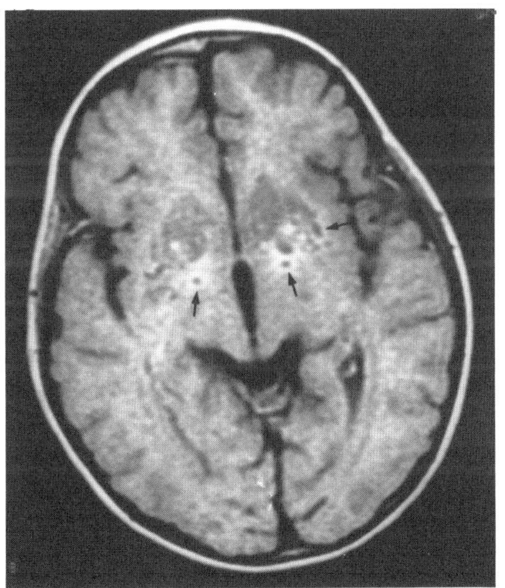

20d

carotid, middle, and anterior cerebral arteries are normal (curved arrow, *c*) (moyamoya disease is excluded). The patient clinically responded well to a steroid therapy. Follow-up (50 days later) T1W image after administration of contrast medium shows apparent regression of the basal ganglia lesions (compare with *a*). However, perivascular enhancement is still seen. Note that the perivascular enhancement (which probably corresponds to inflammatory reaction of the perivascular tissues, a feature of vasculitis) is best appreciated in this image (arrows, *d*).

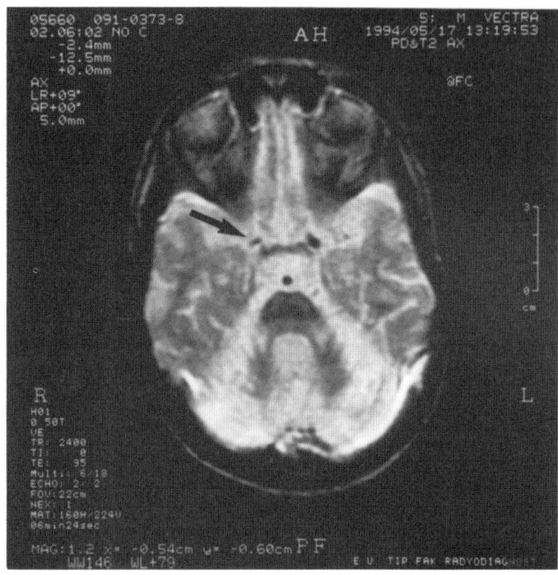

21a

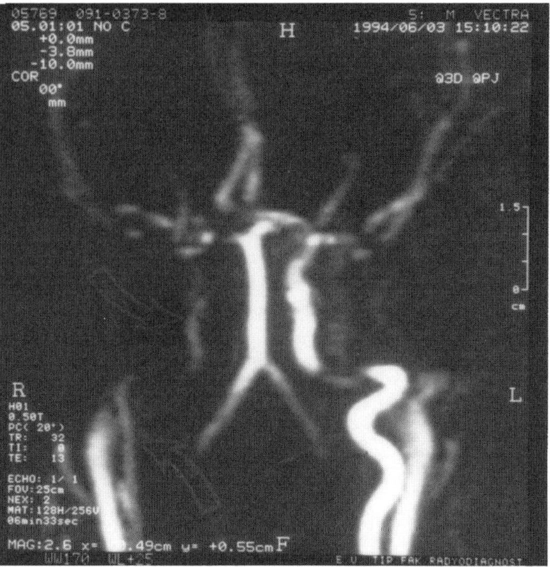

21b

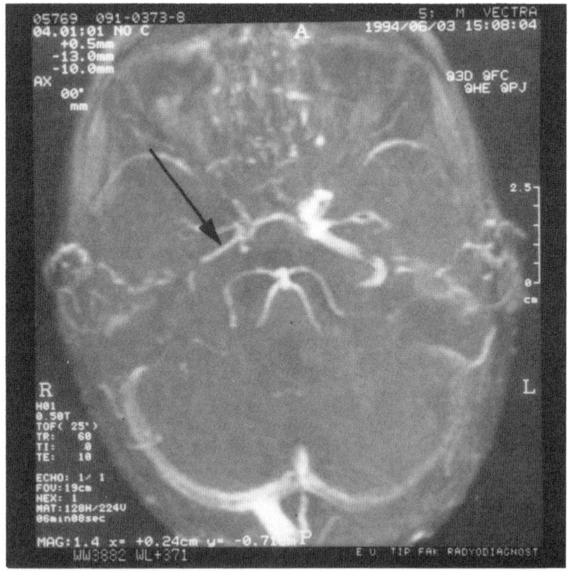

21c

Fig. 21 *a-c. Vasculitis involving the internal carotid artery.* 5-year-old boy. *a,* T2W; *b,* coronal 3D-PC MRA (velocity = 20 cm/sec); and *c,* axial 3D-TOF MRA. T2W image shows that the right internal carotid artery (arrow, *a*) is smaller than the left one. Also, cerebral and cerebellar atrophy is noted. Coronal 3D-PC MRA shows the left internal carotid artery is normal (arrows, *b*). The cervical and cavernous portions of the right internal carotid artery, however, shows apparent narrowing and contour irregularity (open arrows, *b*). 3D-TOF MRA also demonstrates narrowing of the right internal carotid artery (arrow, *c*). The condition was attributed to recurrent nasopharyngeal infections in this patient with mental retardation, after thorough clinical, laboratory, neurologic, and radiologic investigation, which mainly excluded a congenital stenosis of the involved artery, moyamoya disease, and any systemic vascular disease.

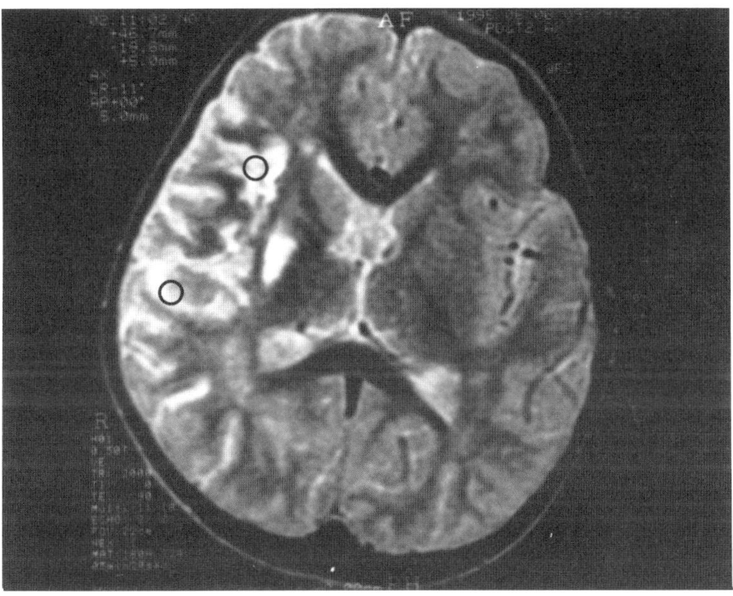

22a

Fig. 22 *a-c. Moyamoya disease.* 3-year-old boy. *a*, axial, T2W; *b*, coronal 3D-PC MRA (velocity = 21cm/sec); and *c*, conventional angiography.

T2W image demonstrates ischemic lesions in the right temporoparietal regions and basal ganglia in this patient with acute neurologic deterioration (*a*). 3D-PC MRA shows a normal intracranial arteries on the left (curved arrow). The right internal carotid artery, however, is narrowed (long arrow), and the right middle cerebral artery is occluded (open arrow) (*b*). Conventional angiography (right carotid injection) verifies these findings, and demonstrates a number of thin, collateral arteries (*c*).

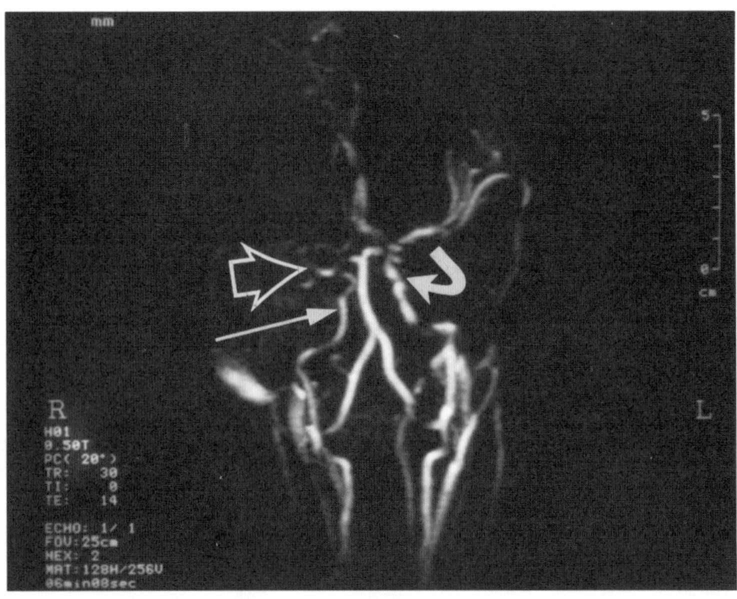

22b

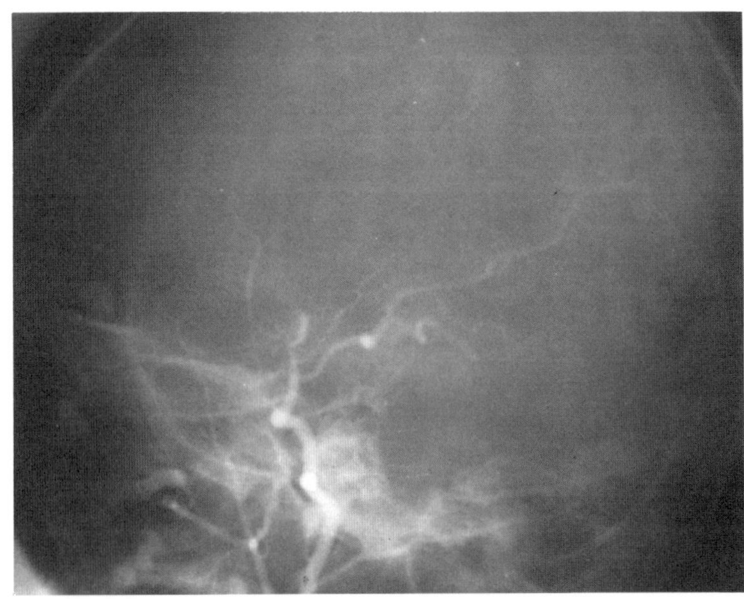

22c

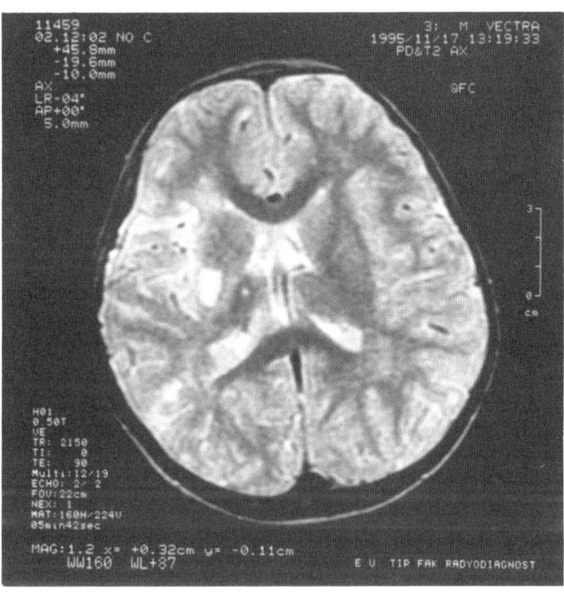

23a

Fig. 23 *a-c. Moyamoya disease after surgical intervention* (5-month follow-up study of the same patient in Fig. 22). The patient had an operation in order to increase the arterial flow to the right hemisphere (encephalodural arteriomyosynangiosis). *a,* T2W, *b,* coronal 3D-PC MRA, and *c,* axial 3D-TOF MRA. T2W image (*a*) shows a chronic ischemic lesion (infarct) in the right putamen, otherwise the other ischemic lesions appear to be resolved (see Fig. 22a). 3D-PC MRA (*b*) shows that the right internal carotid artery is relatively normal (arrows) compared with the previous study (see Fig. 22b). In addition, 3D-TOF MRA (*c*) shows that the right middle cerebral artery is also relatively normal (arrow) compared with its appearance in the previous study (see Fig. 22b), however it is still narrow compared with the contralateral, normal middle cerebral artery. Such improvement of the vascular stenosis is a known feature of moyamoya disease after encephalodural arteriomyosynangiosis.

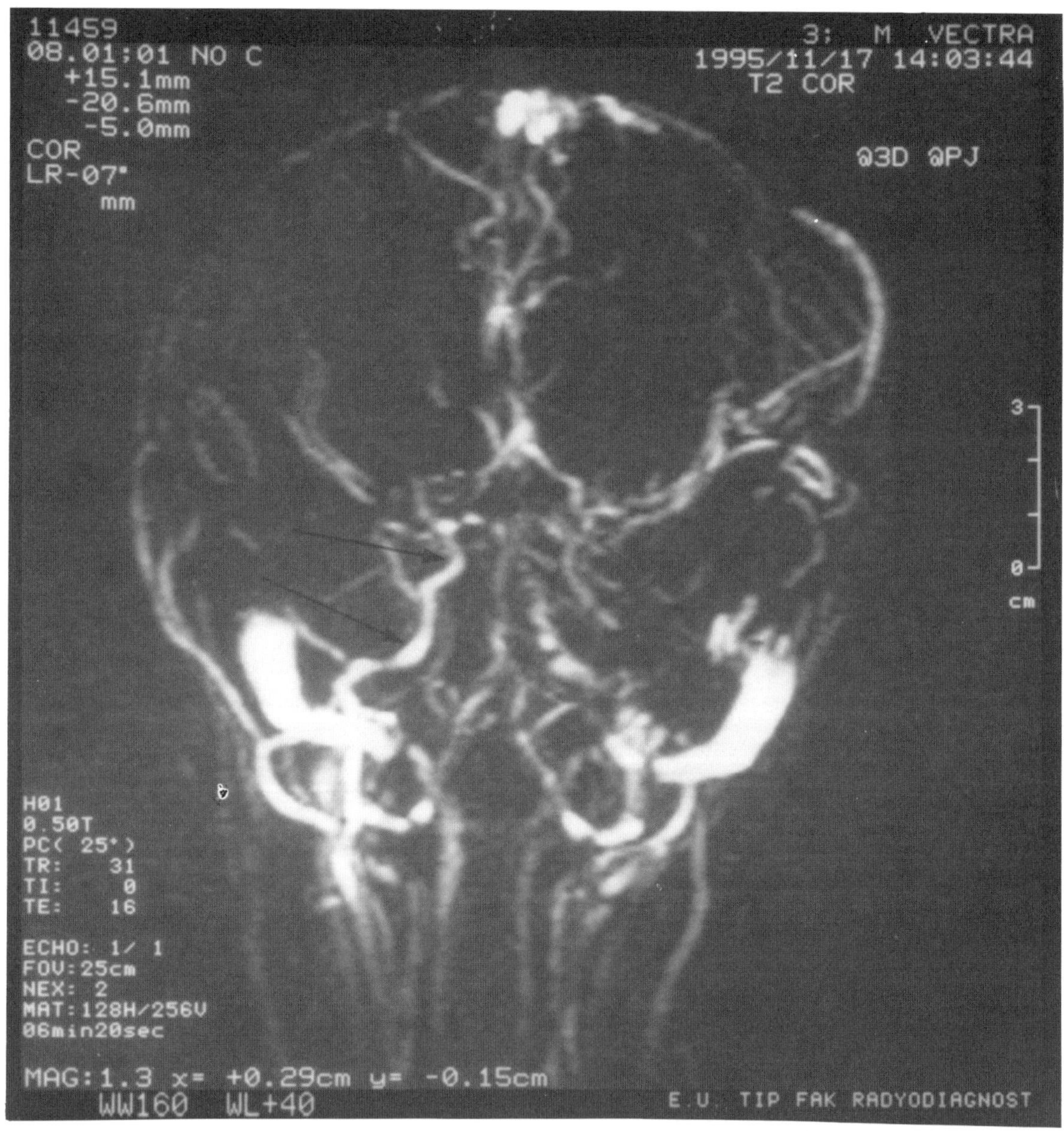

23b

09.01:01 NO C
+31.5mm
-16.0mm
-5.0mm
AX
00°
mm
1995/11/17 14:05:22
T2 COR
@3D @FC
@HE @PJ
3
0
cm
H01
0.50T
TOF(25°)
TR: 60
TI: 0
TE: 10
ECHO: 1/ 1
FOV:19cm
NEX: 1
MAT:128H/224V
06min08sec
MAG:1.1 x= -0.09cm y= -0.20cm
WW334   WL+283
E.U. TIP FAK RADYODIAGNOST

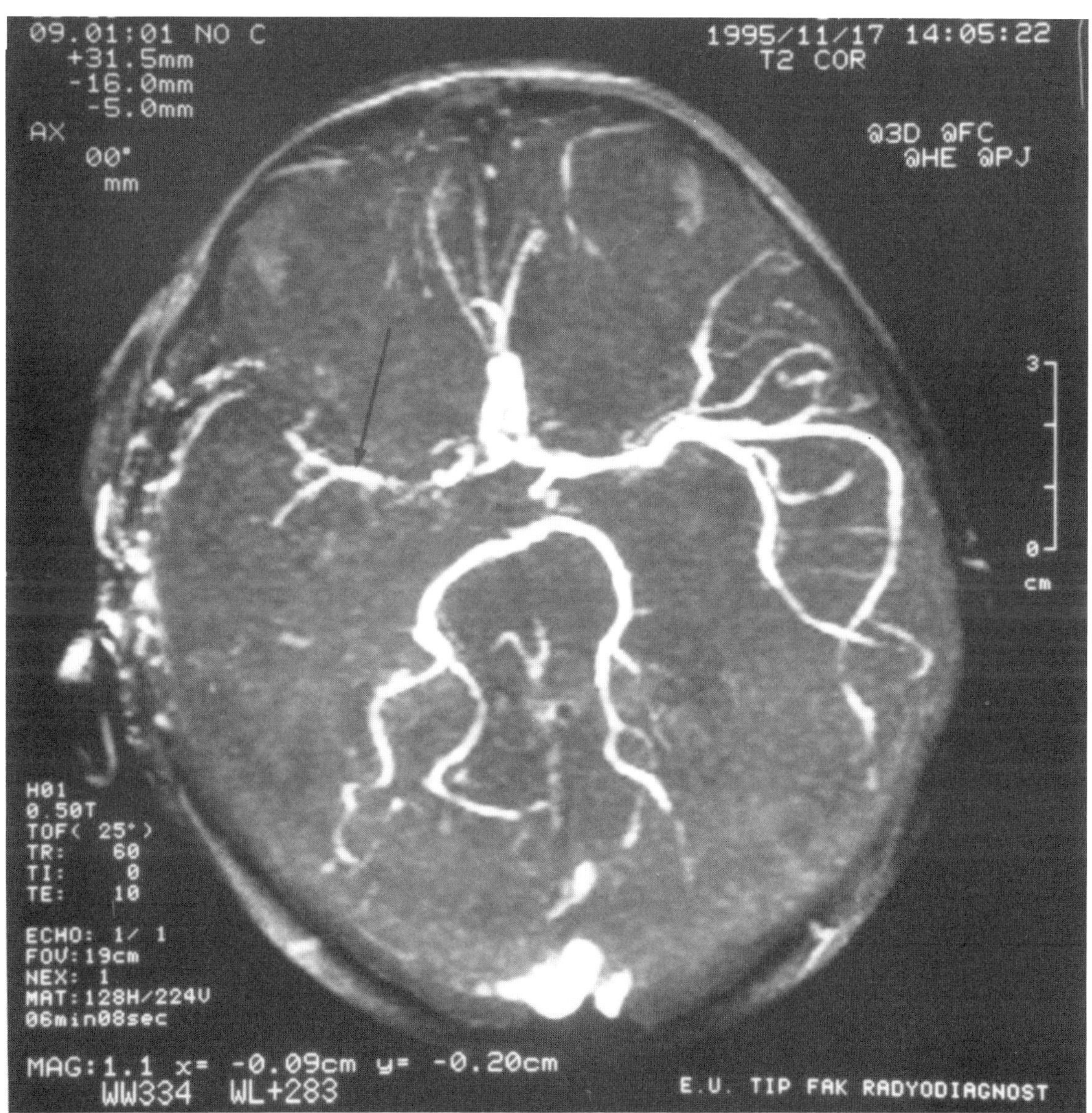

23c

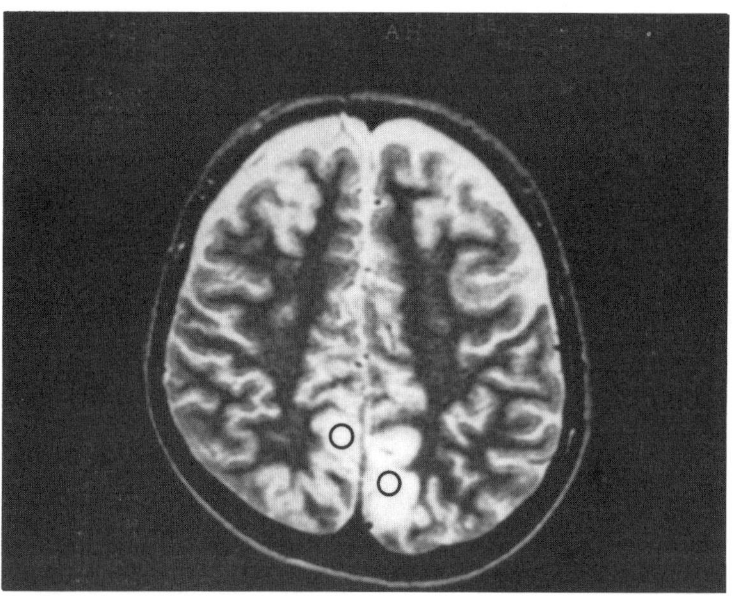

24a

Fig. 24 *a-c. Leukemic vasculopathy.* 9-year-old boy. *a,* axial, T2W; *b,* axial, GRE T1W; and *c,* coronal 3D-PC MRA (velocity = 40cm/sec).

T2W image shows hyperintense lesions in the posterior parietal lobes medially (circles, *a*). GRE, T1W image does not show the normally expected high-signal flow in the middle cerebral arteries (arrows, *b*). The left middle cerebral artery can be identified as a very narrow structure in close inspection (double arrows, *b*). 3D-PC MRA shows that the lumen of the left middle cerebral artery is apparently narrow (arrow on left), and the lumen of the right middle cerebral artery is partly not visualized (arrow on right). These findings have been attributed to a possible spastic reaction of the arteries to the hematologic changes associated with acute lymphoblastic leukemia in this patient (from reference 32).

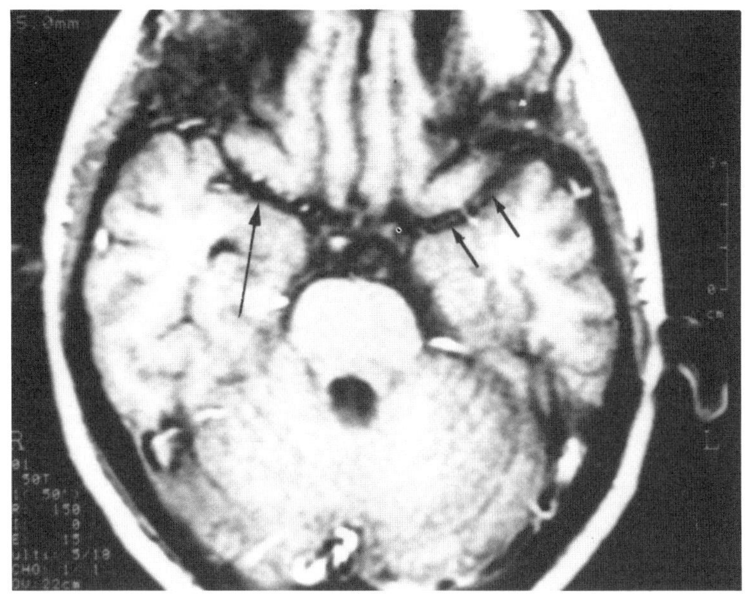

24b

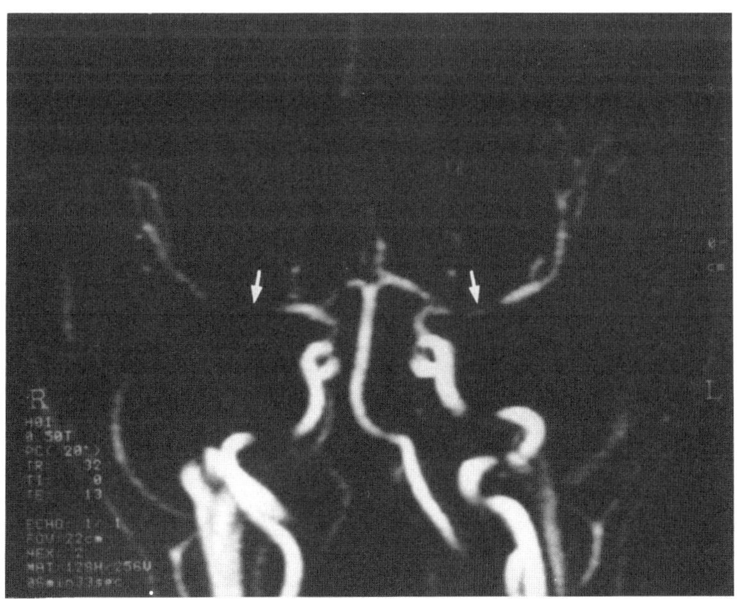

24c

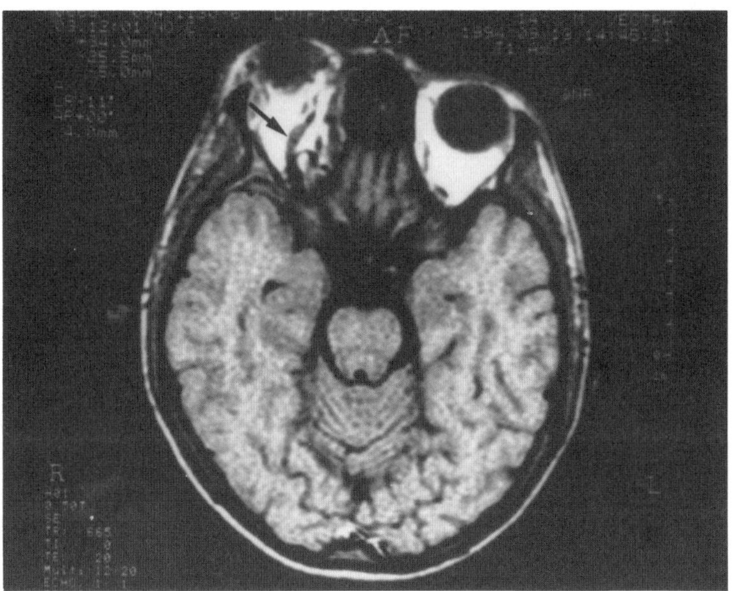

25a

Fig. 25 a-c. *Spontaneous carotid-cavernous fistula in a patient with hemophilia.* 14-year-old boy. *a,* axial, T1W; *b,* axial, 3D-PC MRA (velocity = 20cm/sec); and *c,* sagittal 3D-PC MRA (velocity = 20cm/sec).

T1W image shows right exophthalmus and an enlarged right superior ophthalmic vein (arrow, *a*). 3D-PC MRA's show a direct communication between the right internal carotid artery and right superior ophthalmic vein (arrows, *b,c*). This patient had hemophilia (factor VIII deficiency) and developed this fistula spontaneously.

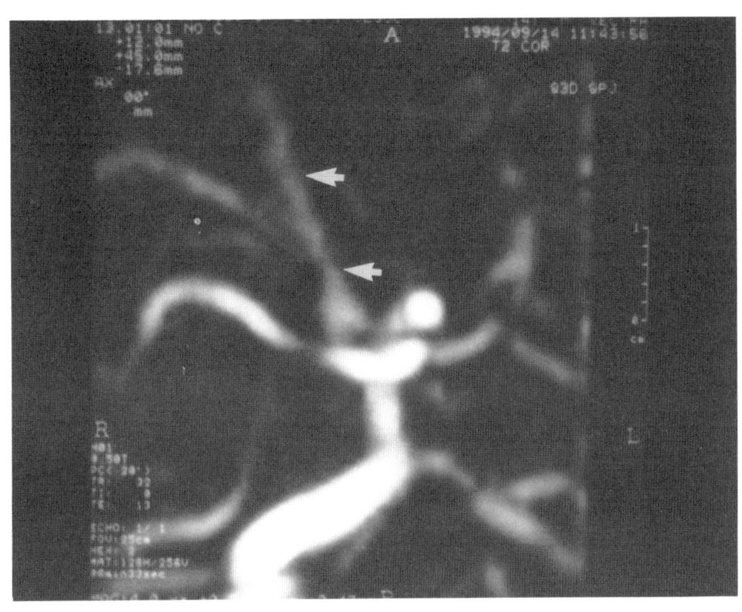

25b

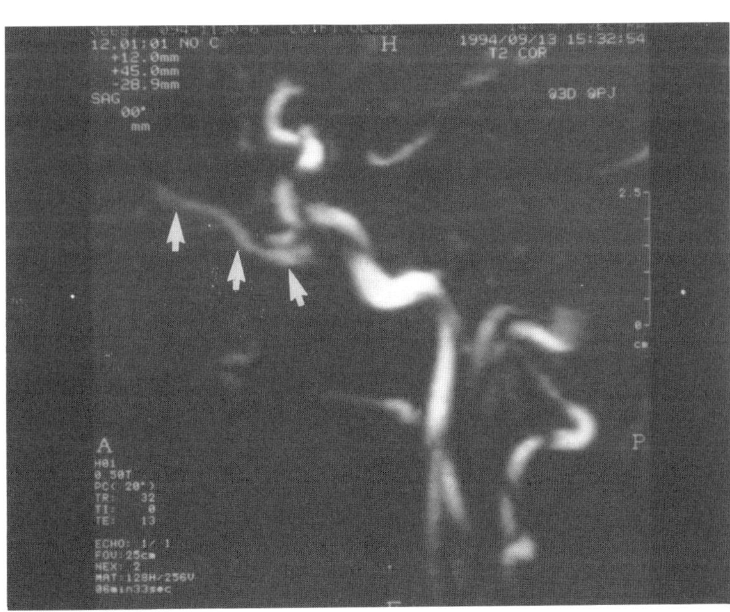

25c

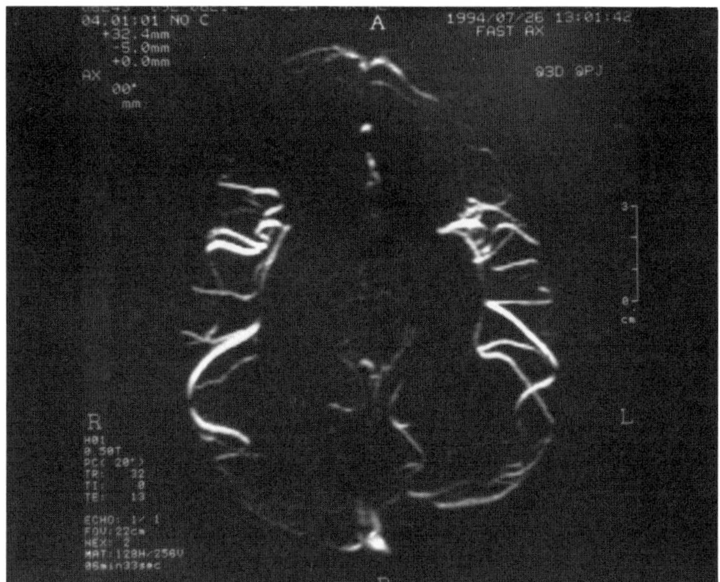

26

Fig. 26 *Normal cortical veins.* 3-year-old boy. 3D-PC MRA (an axial slab of 48mm in thickness centered to the centrum semiovale, velocity = 21cm/sec) shows the appearance of the normal cortical veins (compare this with Fig. 28-33).

Fig. 27 *Normal cortical veins.* 2.5-year-old girl. 3D-TOF MRA (an axial slab of 48mm in thickness centered to the centrum semiovale) shows the normal cortical veins (compare this with Fig. 28-33).

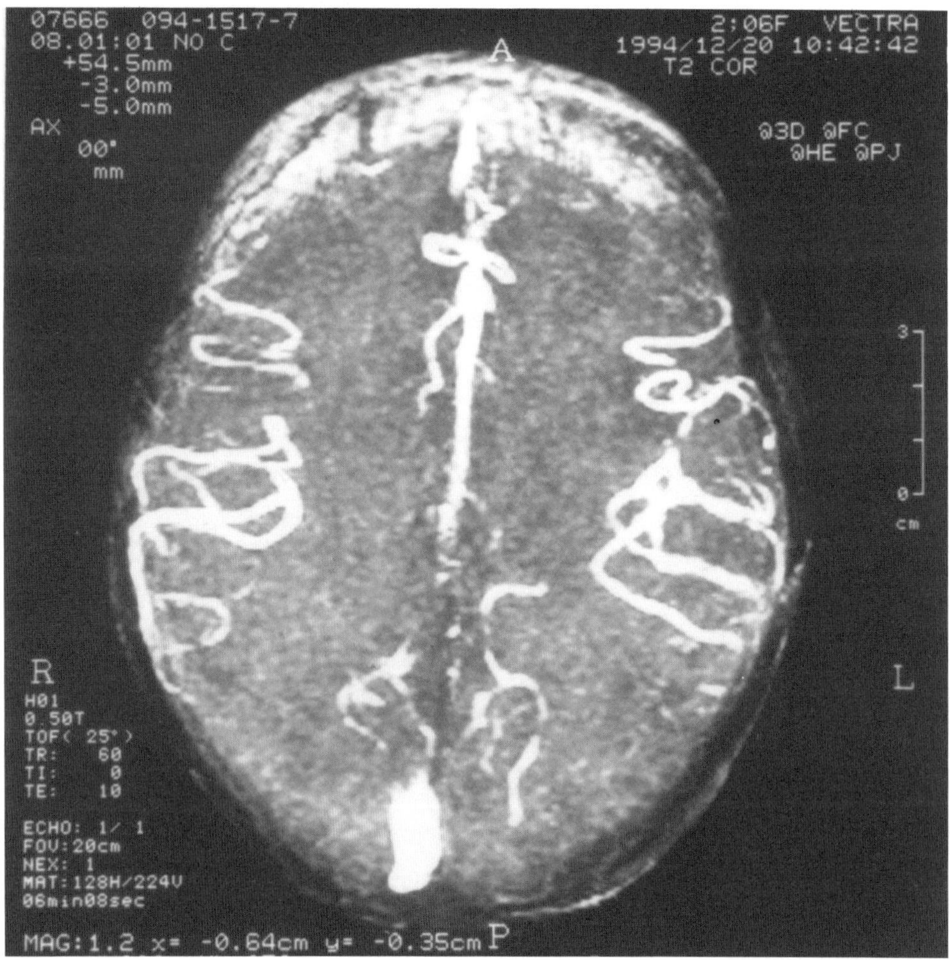

27

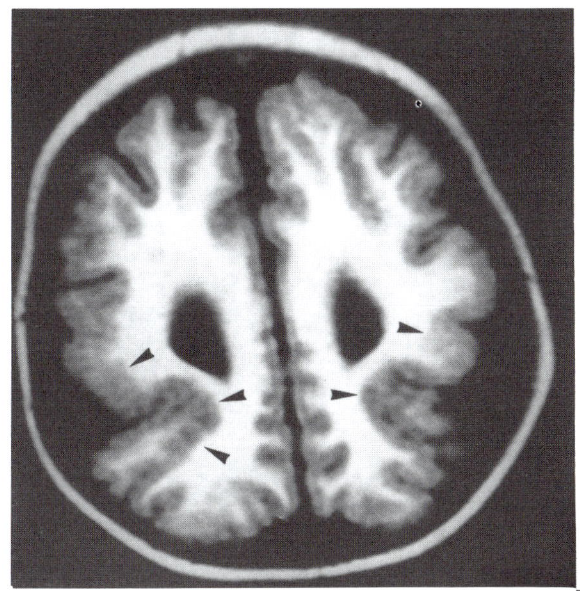

28a

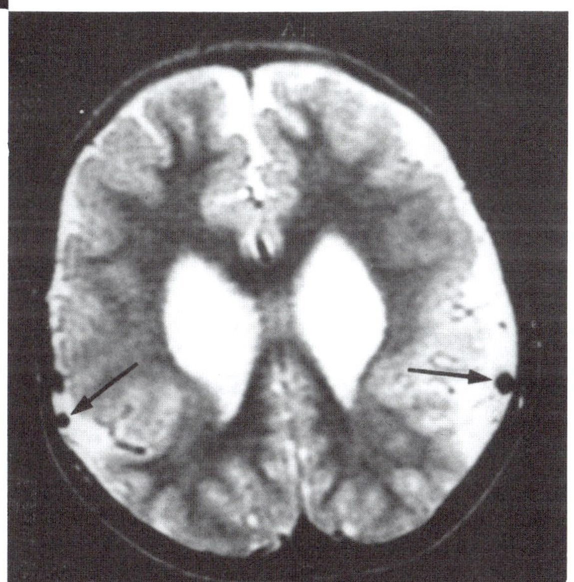

28b

Fig. 28 *a-d*. *Polymicrogyria.* 4-year-old boy. *a,* axial, T1W (inversion recovery); *b,* axial, T2W; *c,* axial, 3D-PC MRA (velocity = 20cm/sec); and *d,* coronal, 3D-PC MRA (velocity = 20cm/sec).

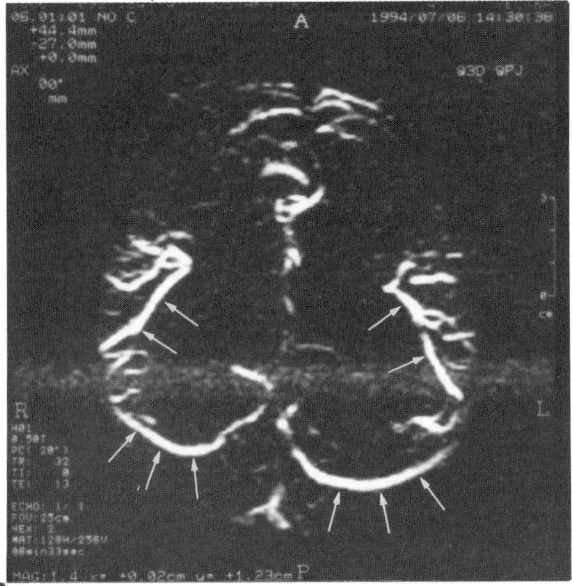

28c

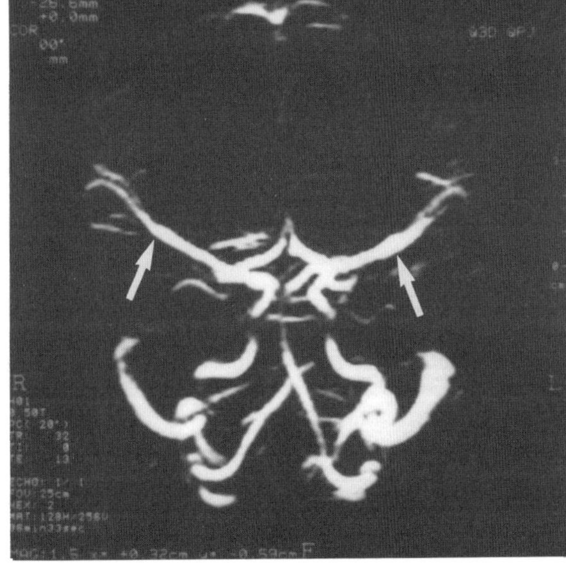

28d

T1W image shows bilateral, thick cortical infoldings and densely packed multiple gyri, consistent with polymicrogyria (arrowheads, *a*). T2W image shows a number of possibly abnormal venous structures (arrows, *b*). 3D-PC MRA in axial projection at the level of centrum semiovale shows abnormal embryonic veins surrounding the abnormal cortices (arrows, c), which frequently accompany neuronal migrational disorders. 3D-PC MRA in coronal projection centered at the level of the circle of Willis, shows abnormally oblique orientation of the middle cerebral arteries (arrows) due to the high position of the sylvian fissures caused by rolandic cortical infoldings (*d*).

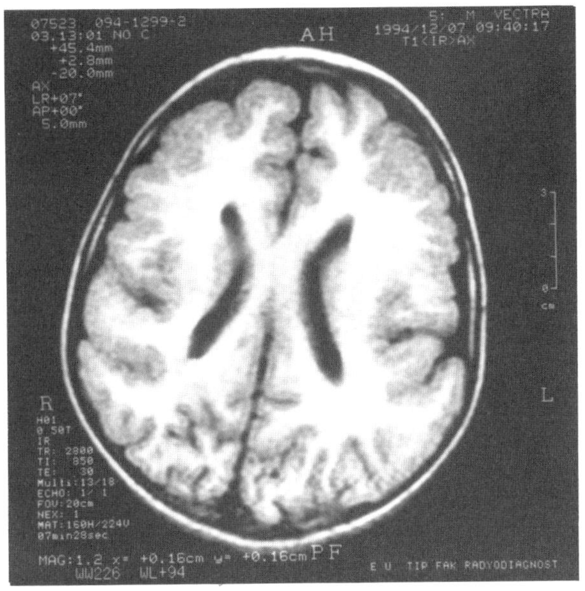

29a

Fig. 29 *a-c. Polymicrogyria.*
5-year-old boy. *a,* axial, T1W (inversion recovery); *b,* and *c,* axial, 3D-PC MRA (MIP reconstructions of 3D-PC MRA at two different planes, velocity = 6 cm/sec). There is diffuse cortical thickening in the frontal and parietal lobes associated with cortical infoldings in the perisylvian and Rolandic regions (*a*), consistent with cortical dysplasia (polymicrogyria). 3D-PC MRA shows the abnormal veins surrounding the abnormal cortices (arrows, *b,c*).

29b

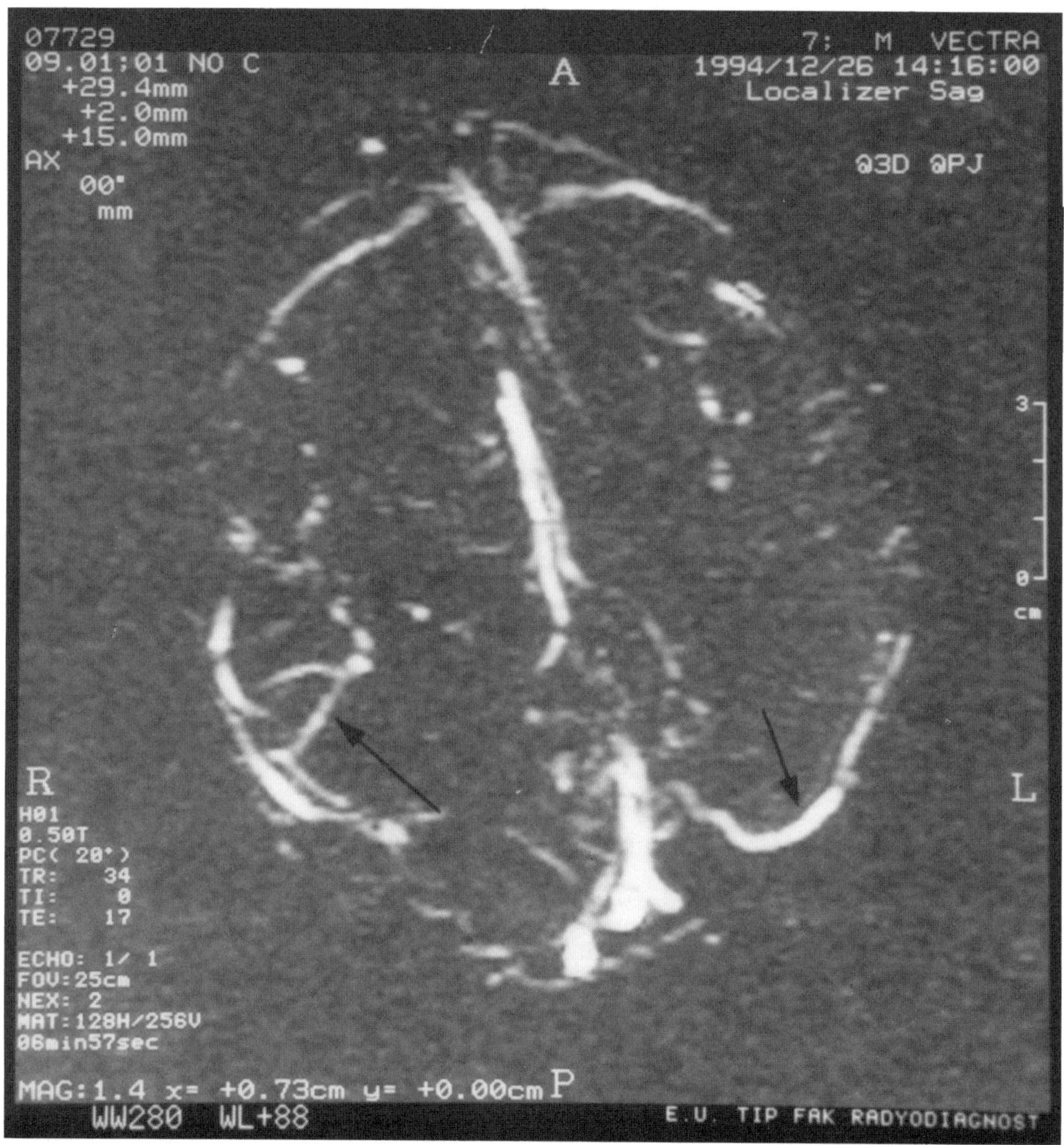

29c

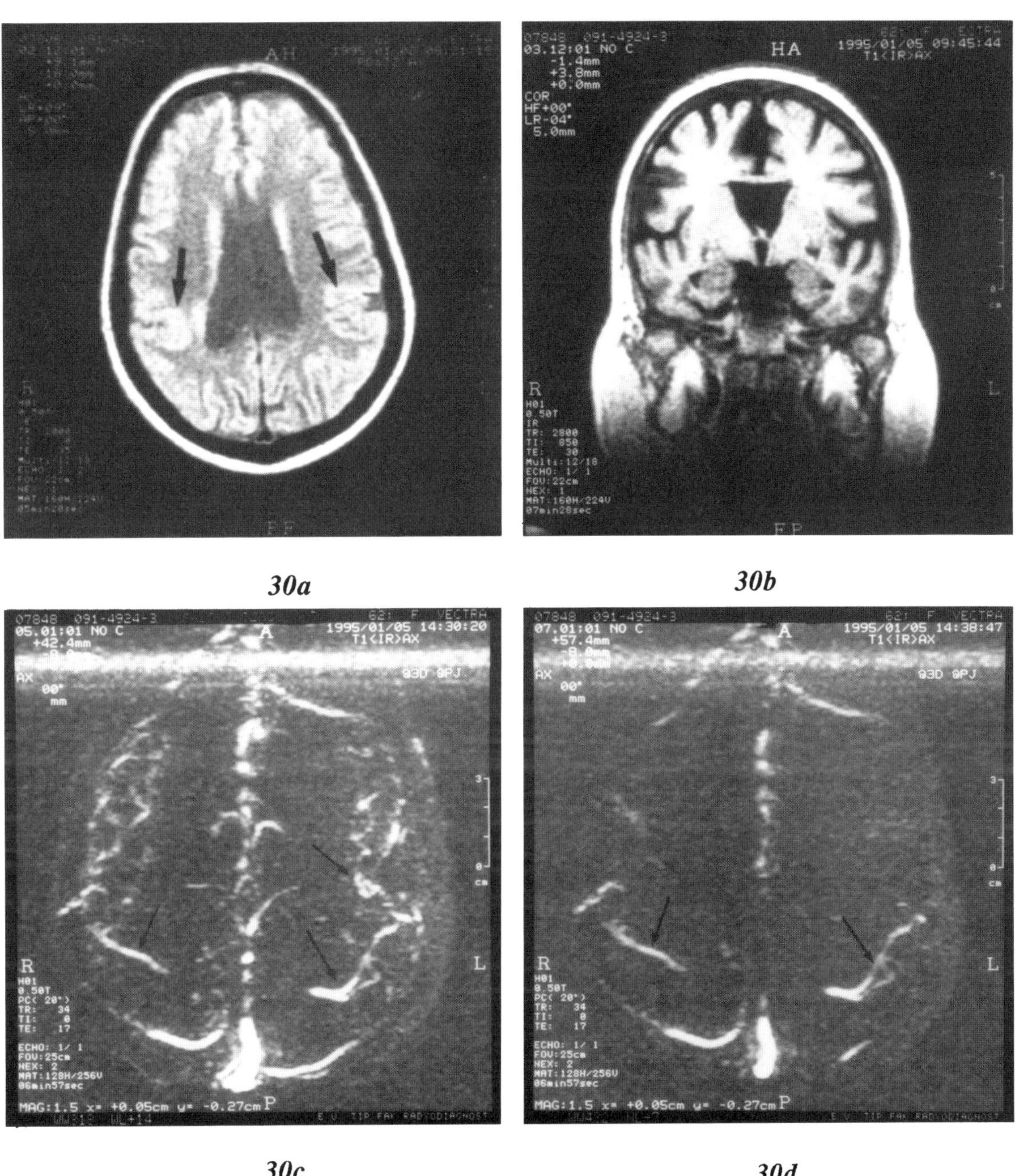

30a   30b

30c   30d

Fig. 30 *a-d. Bilateral cortical dysplasia associated with diffuse atrophy.* 62-year-old woman. *a,* axial PDW; *b,* coronal T1W; *c* and *d,* 3D-PC MRA (MIP reconstructions of 3D-PC MRA at two different planes, velocity = 7 cm/sec). PDW image shows bilateral, thickened cortices and infoldings at the Rolandic regions (arrows, *a*). T1W image reveals diffuse atrophy (*b*).

3D-PC MRA shows abnormal veins surrounding the Rolandic cortices (arrows, *c,d*). Note that the amount of the cortical veins appear to be diminished in this 62-year-old patient also with diffuse atrophy.

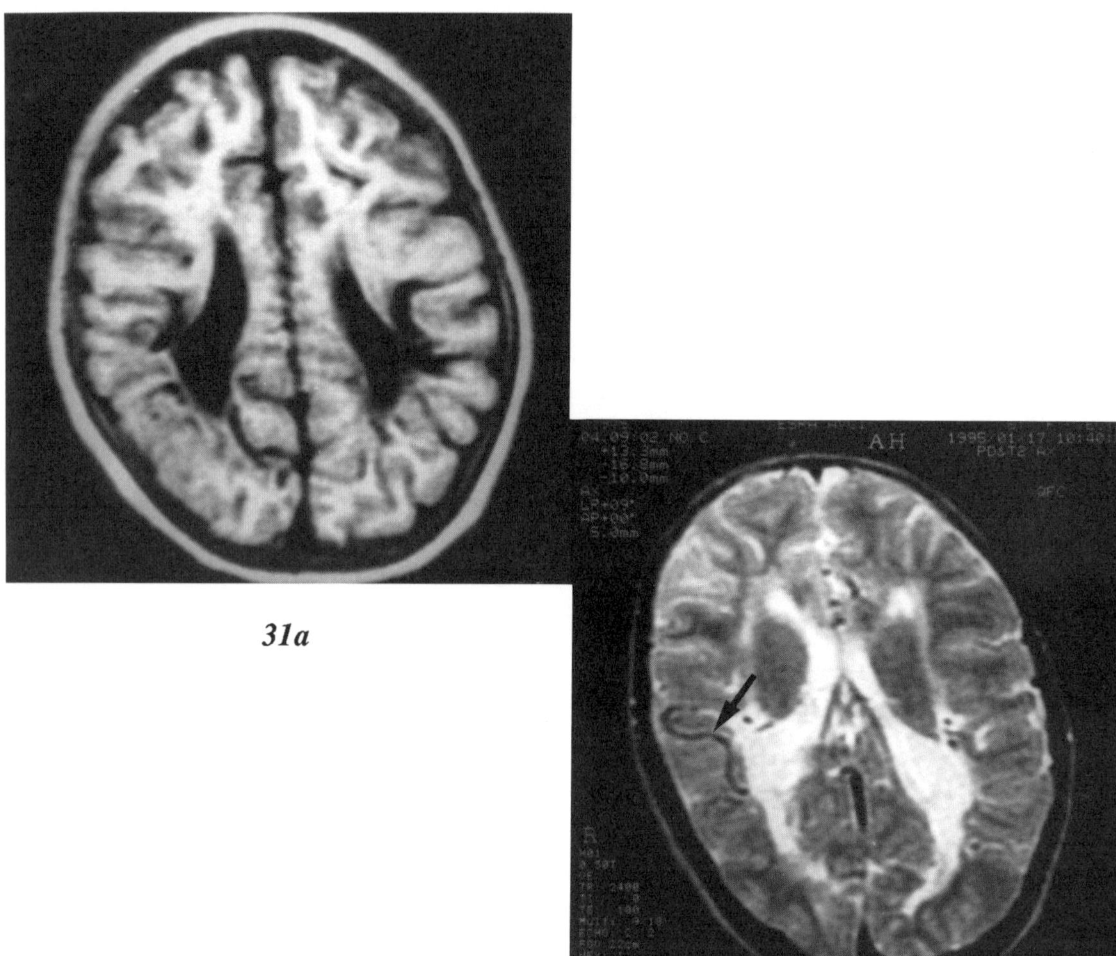

31a

31b

Fig. 31 *a-c. Periventricular leukomalacia.* 8-year-old girl. *a,* axial, T1W; *b,* axial, T2W; and *c,* axial, 3D-PC MRA (velocity = 6cm/sec).

T1W image shows bilateral, periventricular encephaloclastic-gliotic changes, consistent with periventricular leukomalacia (*a*). T2W image shows hyperintense changes in the corresponding regions, and a prominent vessel (vein) with an abnormal course (arrow, *b*). 3D-PC MRA shows prominent, abnormal draining veins in both hemispheres (arrows, *c*) (compare with Fig. 26, 27). In a recent study conducted by us in patients with periventricular leukomalacia, we usually noted a single prominent abnormal vein within the affected hemisphere. Although the reason for this appears to be unclear, we speculate that during the perinatal ischemic episode and subsequent volume loss and gliosis, in the affected region most of the cortical veins become collapsed (and obstructed), leaving behind a few normal ones, and consequently one (or more) of which becomes slightly thickened, and elongated to enable effective venous drainage from the region (from reference 34).

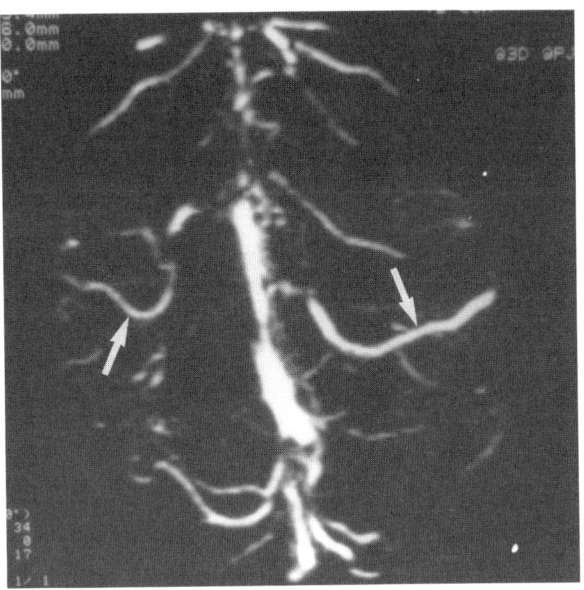

31c

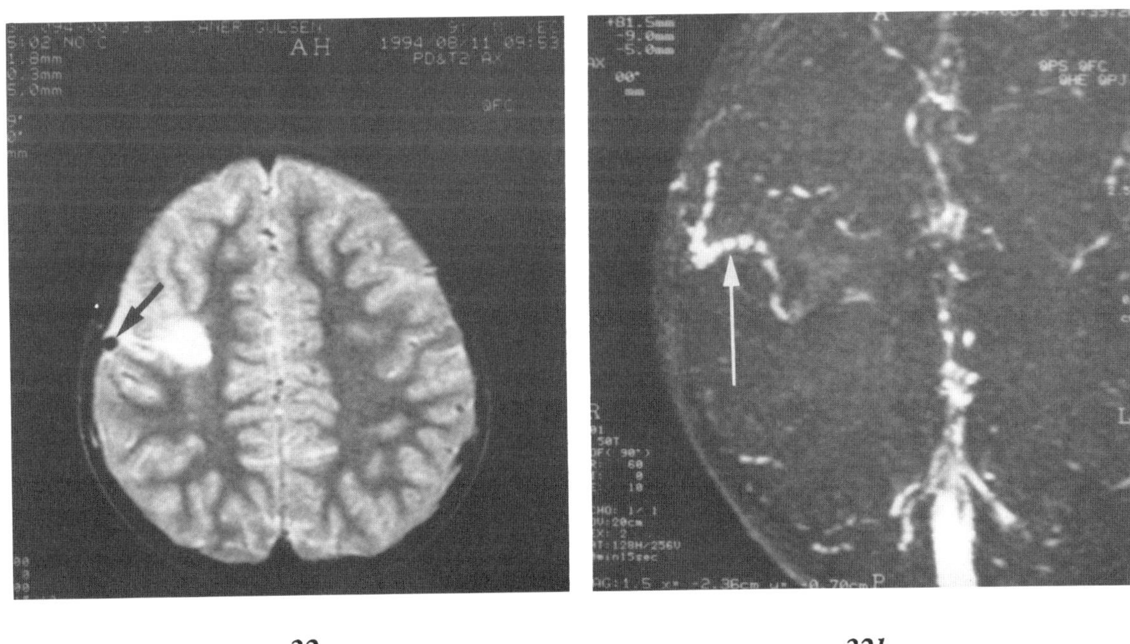

32a   *32b*

Fig. 32 *a,b*. *Periventricular leukomalacia*. 9-year-old boy. *a,* axial, T2W; *b,* axial, 2D-TOF MRA.

    T2W image shows a gliotic region in the right posterior frontal lobe, consistent with periventricular leukomalacia. Note an abnormal vein (arrow, *a*). 2D-TOF MRA shows the abnormal vein (thick, and has an abnormal course) at the corresponding region (arrow, *b*) (compare with Fig. 26, 27).

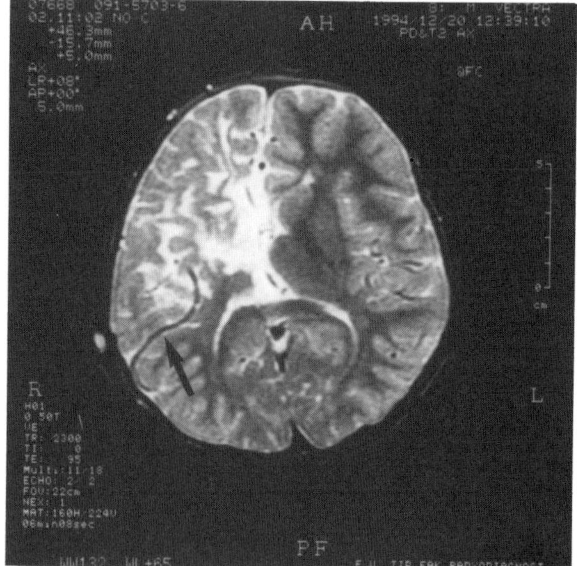

33a

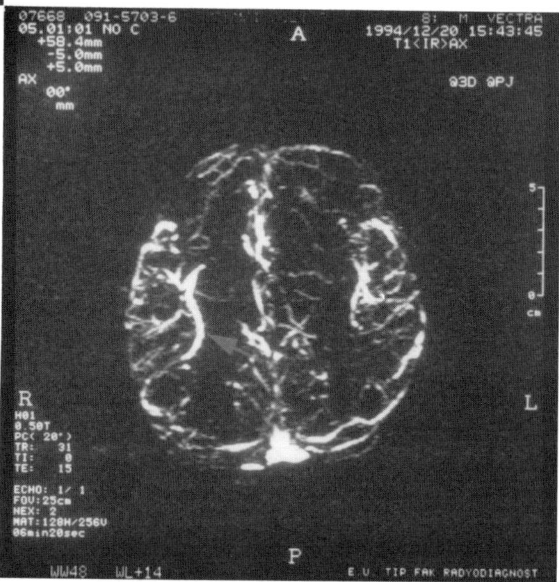

33b

Fig. 33 *a,b*. *Periventricular leukomalacia*. 8-year-old boy. *a,* axial, T2W; and *b,* axial, 3D-PC MRA (velocity = 20cm/sec). T2W image shows extensive gliotic changes in the right hemisphere due to periventricular leukomalacia, and a prominent draining vein (arrow, a). 3D-PC MRA shows the abnormal vein (arrow, b) (compare with Fig. 26, 27).

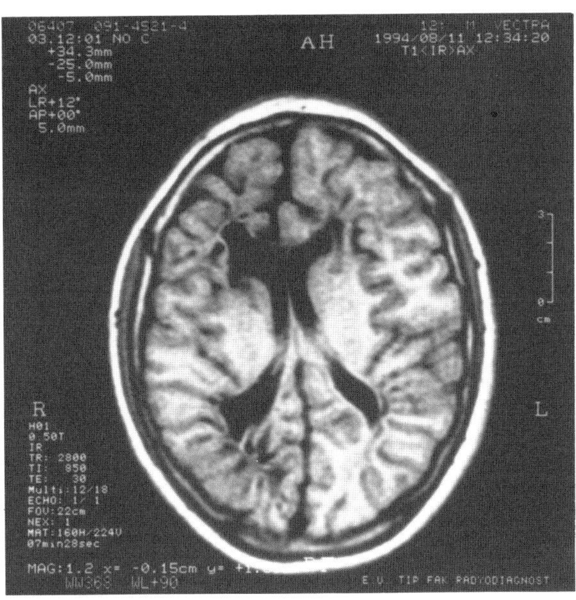

34a

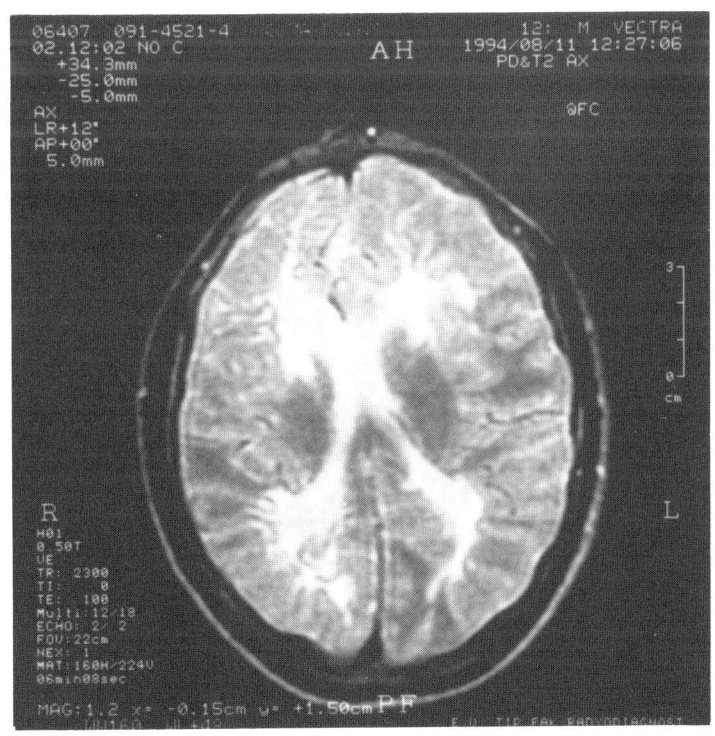

Fig. 34 *a-d. Thinned middle cerebral arteries in bilateral periventricular leukomalacia.* 12-year-old boy. *a,* axial T1W (inversion recovery); *b,* axial T2W; *c,* 3D-TOF MRA; and *d,* 2D-TOF MRA. There is extensive gliosis in both hemispheres due to periventricular leukomalacia *(a,b).* 3D-TOF MRA shows apparent thinning of the middle cerebral arteries (arrows, *c*), which is confirmed by the 2D-TOF MRA (arrows, *d*) (compare with Fig. 35).

34b

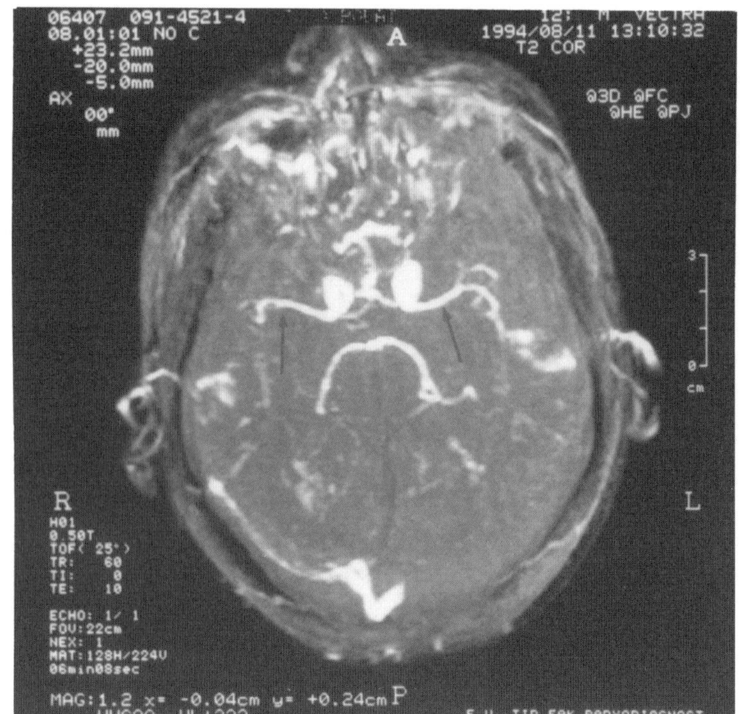

34c

34d

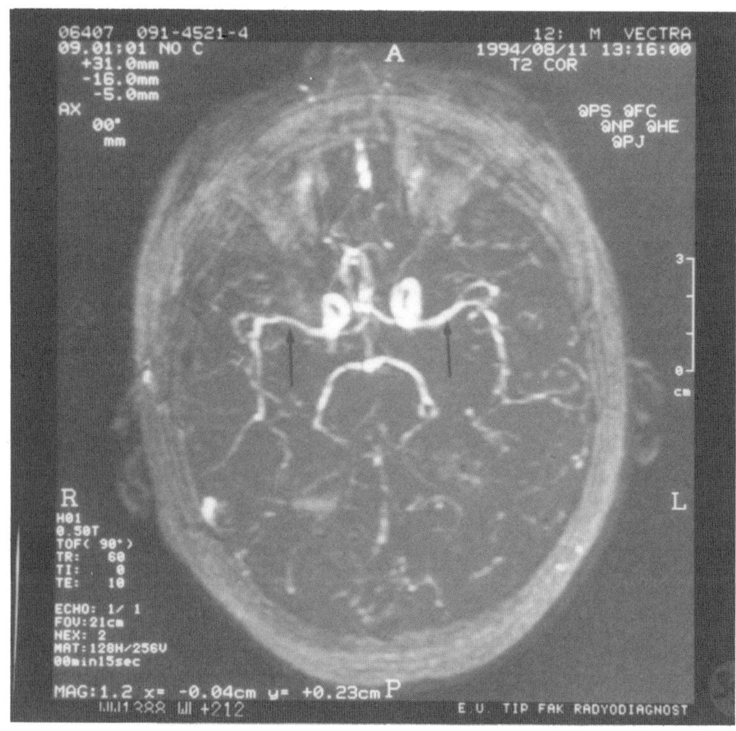

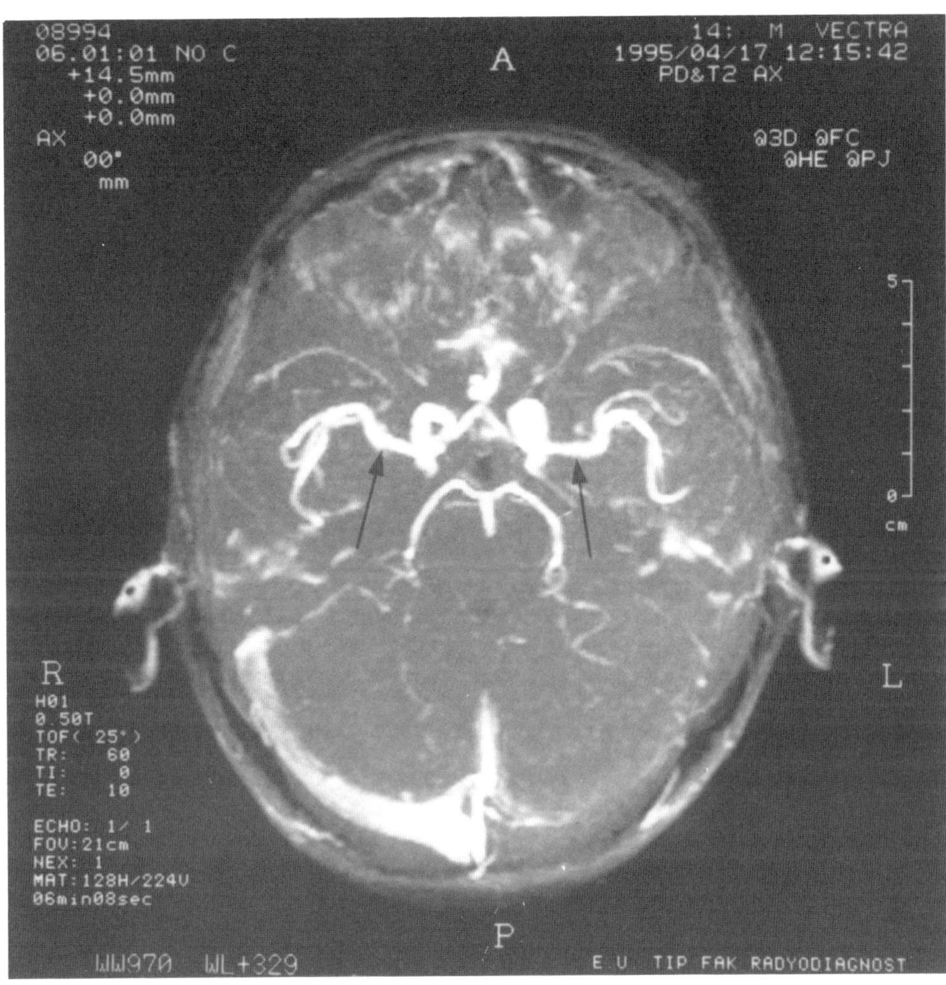

35a

Fig. 35 *a,b*. *Normal middle cerebral arteries*. Age-matched (14-year-old normal boy)
to the patient in Fig. 34. *a,* 3D-TOF MRA, a 48 mm slab centered at the level of the polygon
of Willis; and *b,* 3D-TOF MRA a 48 mm slab centered right above the former level. Note the
appearance of the normal middle cerebral arteries (arrows, *a,b*) (compare with Fig. 34).

08994
11.01:01 NO C
+25.0mm
+0.0mm
+0.0mm
AX
00°
mm
A
14: M VECTRA
1995/04/17 13:42:48
PD&T2 AX
@3D @FC
@HE @PJ
R
H01
0.50T
TOF(25°)
TR: 60
TI: 0
TE: 10
ECHO: 1/ 1
FOV:21cm
NEX: 1
MAT:128H/224V
06min08sec
L
P
WW766 WL+322
E.U. TIP FAK RADYODIAGNOST

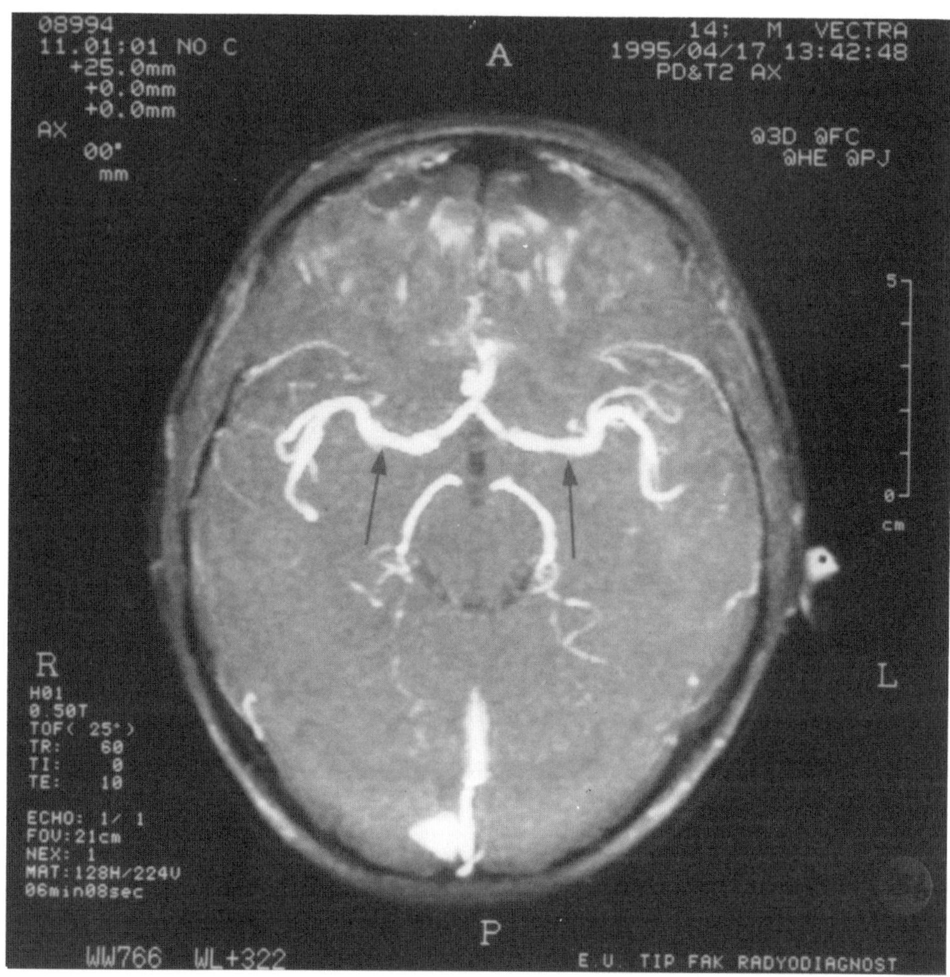

35b

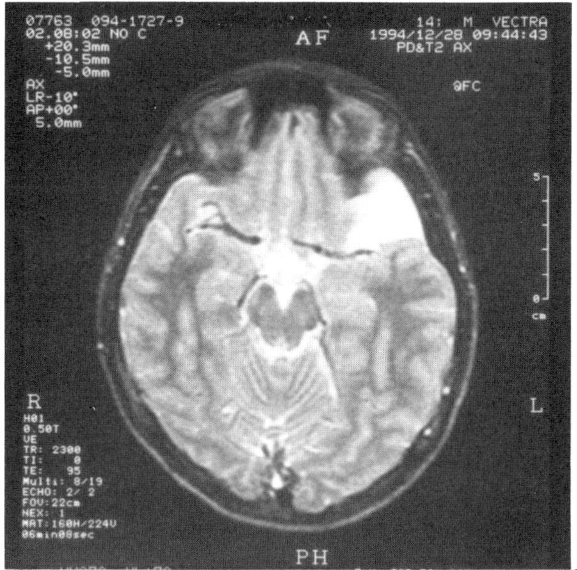

36a

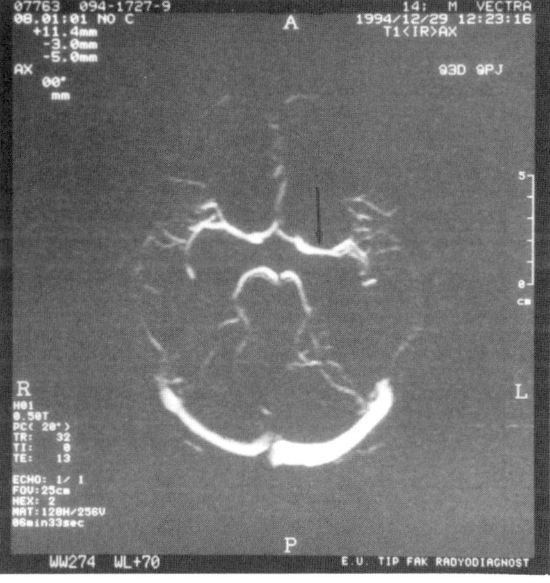

36b

Fig. 36 *a,b*. *Temporal fossa arachnoid cyst.* 14-year-old boy. *a,* axial T2W; and *b,* axial 3D-PC MRA. There is an arachnoid cyst in the left temporal fossa, which displaces the middle cerebral artery posteriorly (*a*), which is confirmed by the 3D-PC MRA (arrow, *b*). This can be a useful sign in discriminating a small temporal fossa arachnoid cyst from temporal lobe hypogenesis, as an arachnoid cyst is expected to produce a compression effect upon the surrounding vessels, while in temporal lobe hypogenesis this finding should not be seen. This is clinically significant, especially because temporal lobe hypogenesis or agenesis is known to be associated with certain metabolic disorders such as glutaric aciduria Type I.

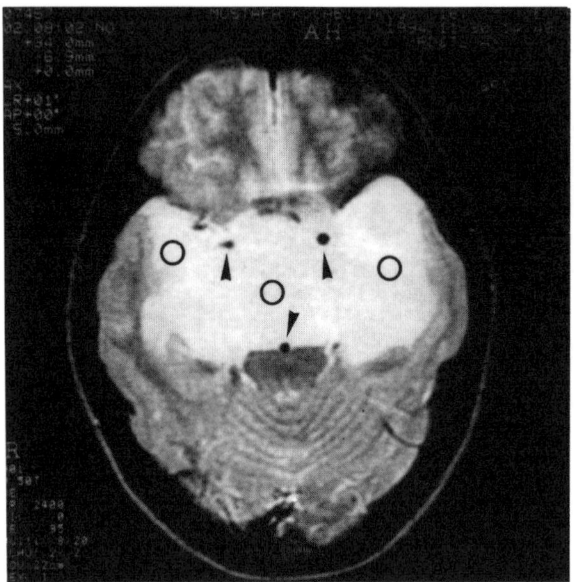

37a

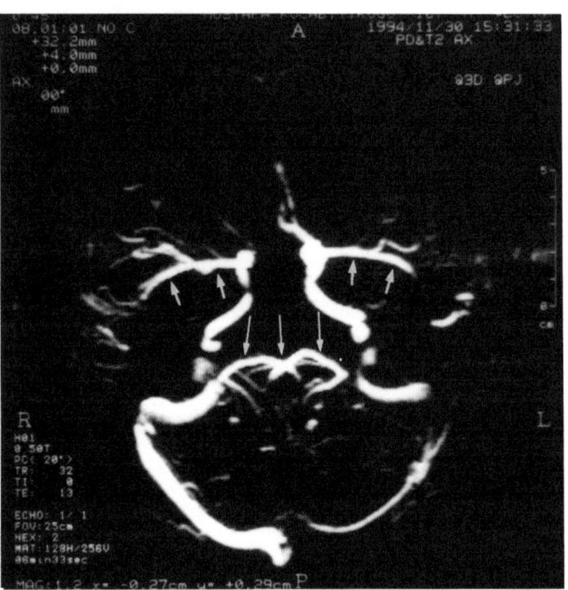

37b

Fig. 37 *a,b. Giant, trilobated arachnoid cyst*. 16-year-old boy. *a,* axial, T2W; and *b,* axial, 3D-PC MRA (velocity=21cm/sec).

T2W image shows a giant trilobated arachnoid cyst with extensions to both temporal regions and suprasellar region (circles, *a*). Displacement of major vessels readily noted (arrowheads, *a*). 3D-PC MRA shows apparent displacement of vessels (middle cerebral arteries, vertebral and basilar arteries) to best advantage (arrows, *b*).

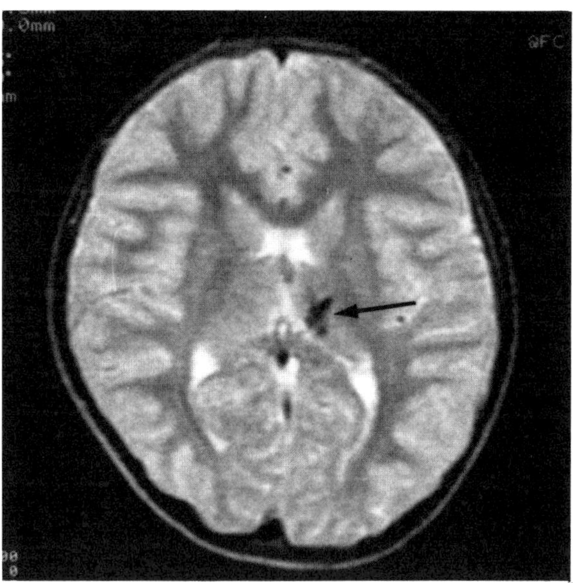

38a

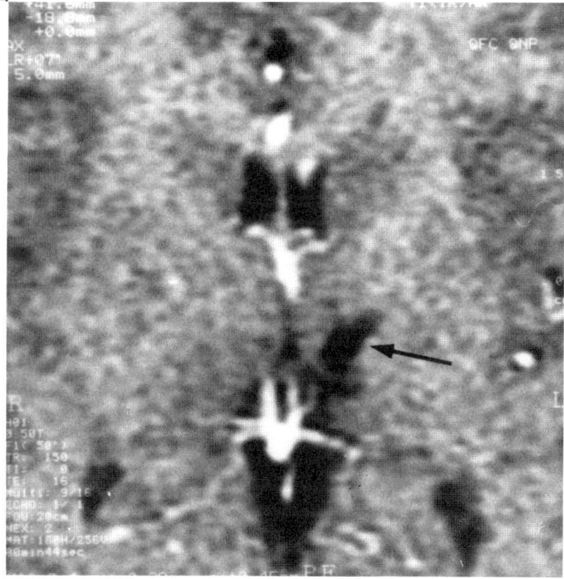

38b

Fig. 38 *a-d. Cavernous angioma.* 7-year-old girl. *a,* axial, T2W; *b,* axial, GRE T1W; *c,* axial, 2D-TOF MRA; and *d,* axial 3D-TOF MRA.

T2W image shows an amorphous hypointensity in the left thalamus (arrow, *a*). GRE, T1W image shows diffuse hypointensity of the lesion, reflecting the magnetic susceptibility effect of hemorrhage (arrow, *b*), and no abnormal vessel is seen excluding an arteriovenous malformation. 2D-TOF MRA shows the lesion to be hypointense (arrow, *c*). 3D-TOF MRA shows the lesion as a hyperintense structure (arrow, *d*). This discrepancy between the two TOF angiograms suggest direct visualization of the vascular lesion (cavernous angioma) on this 3D-TOF angiogram (*d*) (see text).

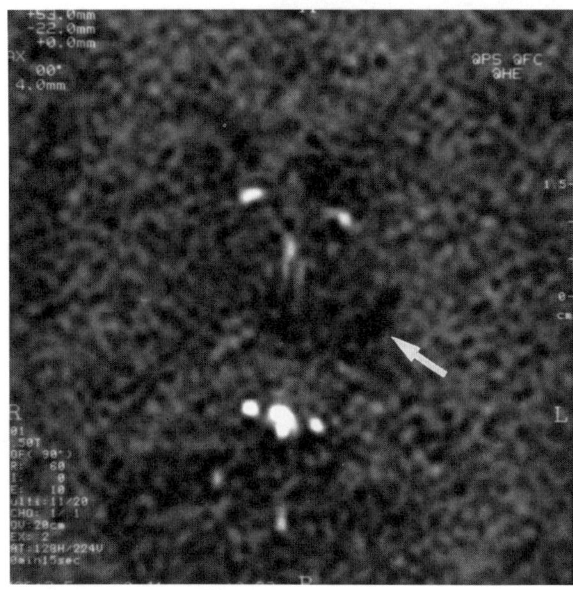

38c

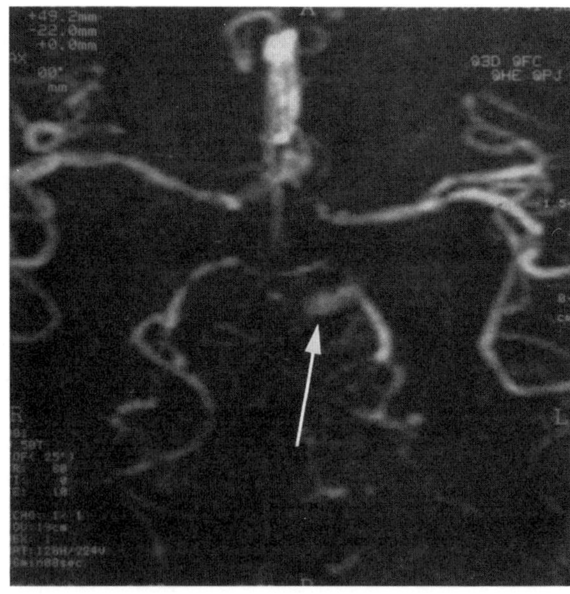

38d

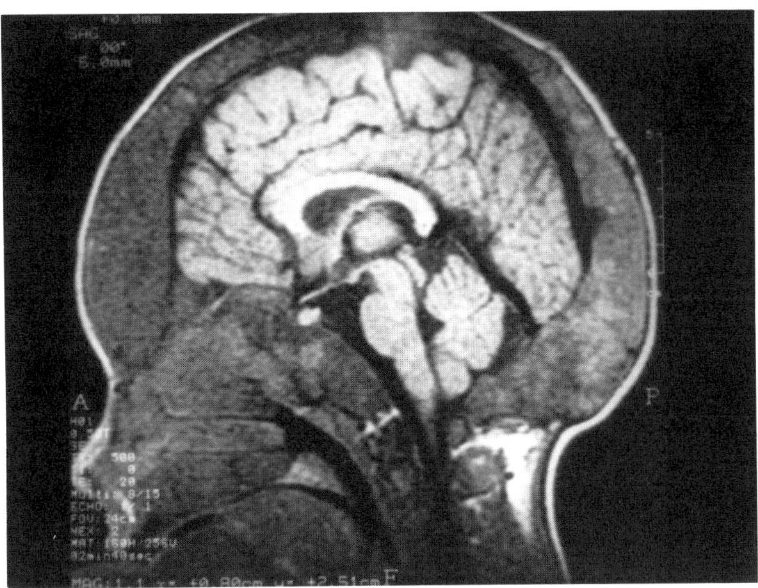

39a

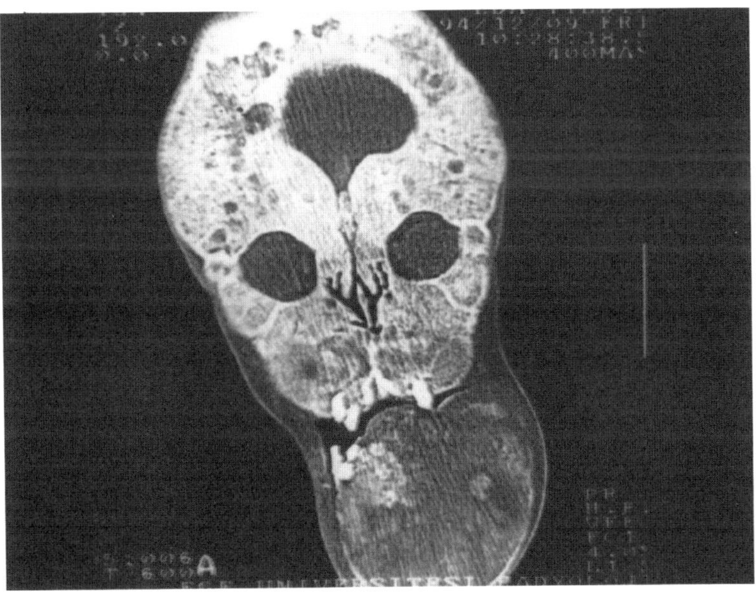

39b

Fig. 39 *a-d*. *Fibrous dysplasia.* 11-year-old girl. *a,* sagittal, T1W; *b,* coronal, CT scan; *c,* coronal, 3D-PC MRA (velocity = 20cm/sec), and *d,* axial, 3D-TOF MRA. T1W image shows extensive cranial changes secondary to fibrous dysplasia (*a*). Note the CT appearance of the extensive lesion (*b*). 3D-PC MRA (*c*) and 3D-TOF MRA (*d*) show prominent extracranial vessels (external carotid artery branches and superficial veins (large arrows, *c*). A number of vessels traverse the thickened calvarium (small arrows, *c, d*). Intracranial vessels appear normal (*c,d*).

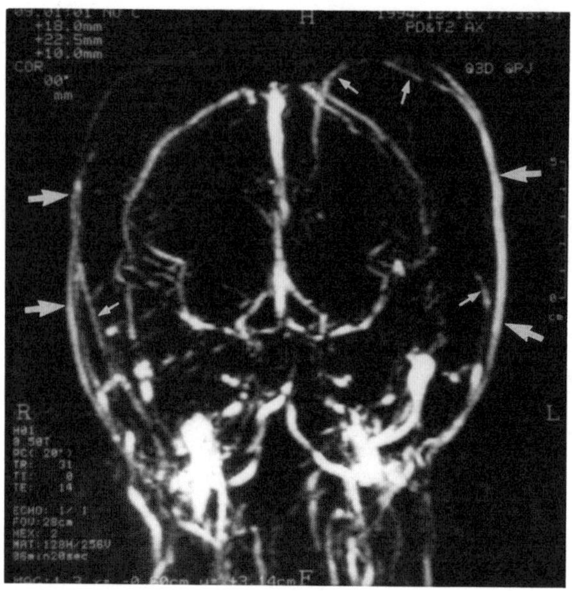

39c

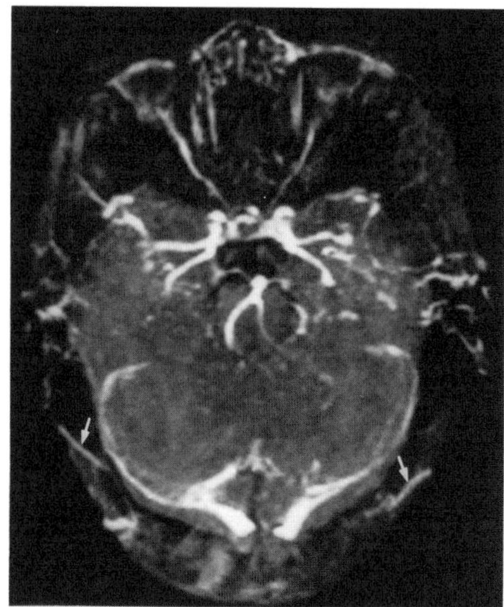

39d

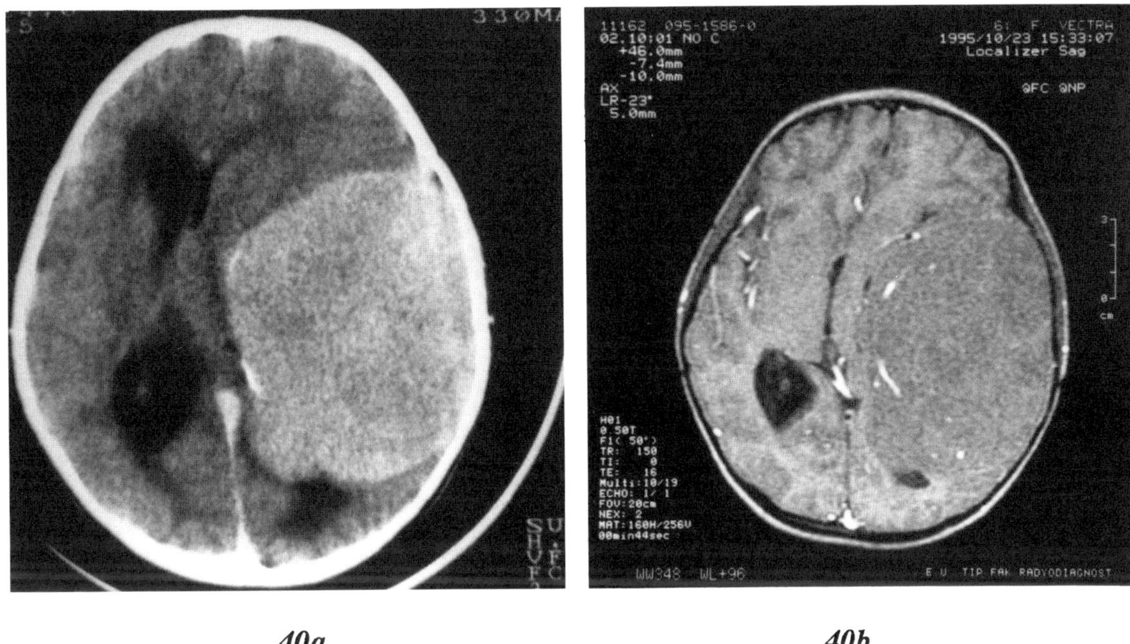

40a   40b

Fig. 40 *a-h.* ***Large meningioma.*** 6-year-old girl. *a,* axial CT scan; *b,* axial GRE T1W; *c,* axial PDW; *d,* axial T2W; *e,* axial T1W after administration of contrast medium; *f,* coronal T1W after administration of contrast medium; *g,* axial 3D-TOF MRA; and *h,* coronal 3D-PC MRA. CT scan shows a large mass with high density in the left hemisphere, and a gross distortion of the brain anatomy with a left-to-right shift (*a*). The mass has a grossly isointense signal to the brain cortex throughout the MR imaging sequences, suggesting a tumor tissue with a high nuclear/cytoplasmic ratio (*b-d*). T2W image, however, shows a relatively inhomogeneous appearance, reflecting calcific and edematous tissue within the tumor (*d*). The images after administration of contrast medium show intense enhancement of the tumor, along with intratumoral vessels and nonenhancing foci. These also show the close proximity of the tumor with the calvarium without an intervening brain tissue, suggesting that the lesion is extra-axial (*e, f*). 3D-TOF MRA, and 3D-PC MRA clearly show displacement of the left middle cerebral artery (long arrows, *g, h*), and its branches supplying the meningioma (short arrows, *g, h*).

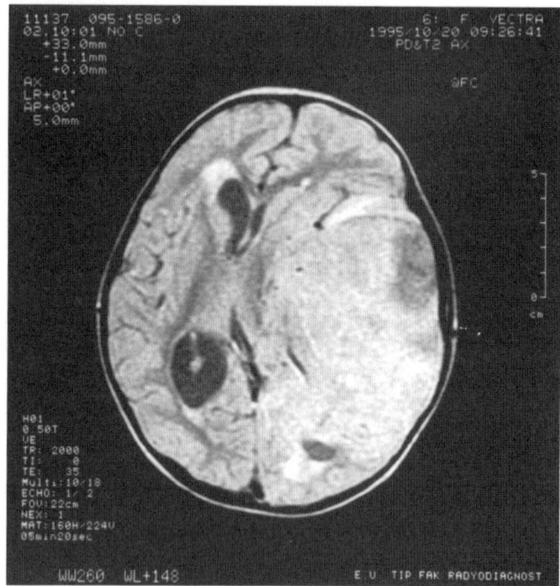

40c

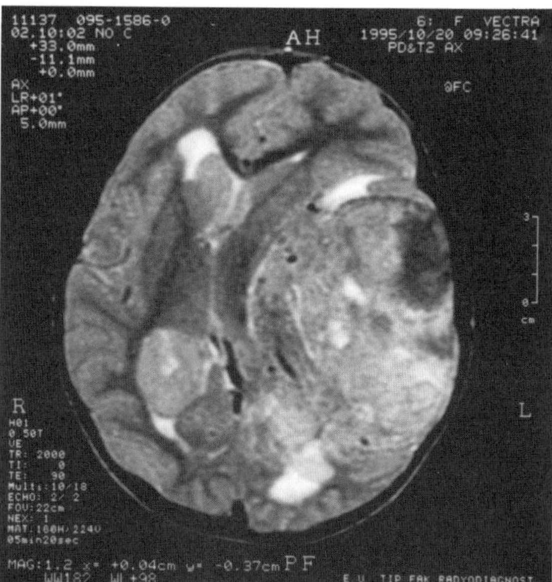

40d

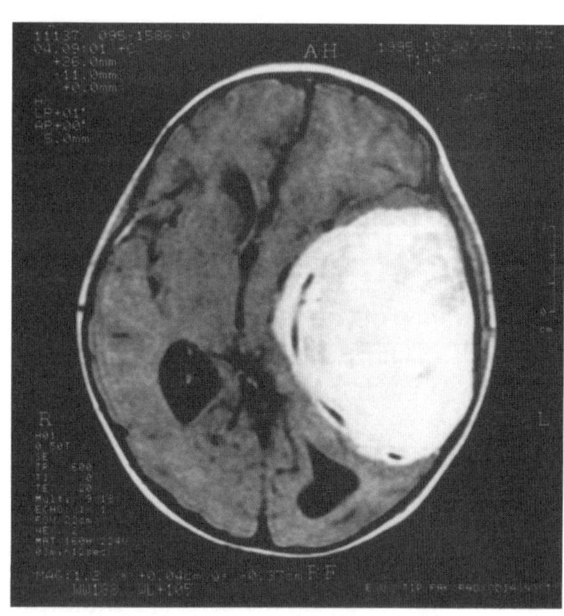

40e

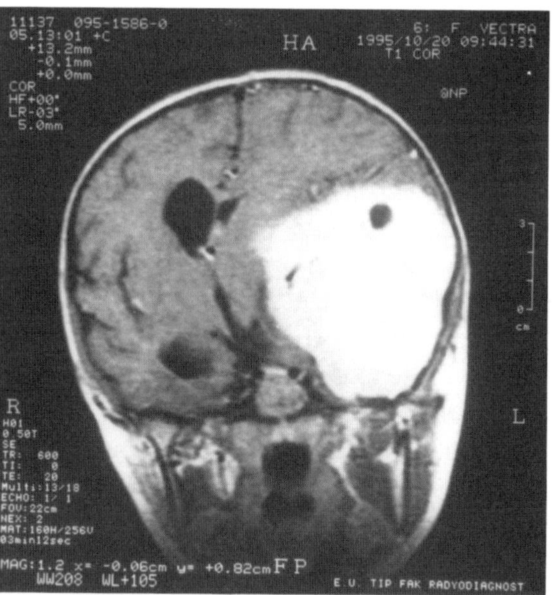

40f

11162 095-1586-0
12.01:01 NO C
+46.3mm
-10.0mm
-5.0mm
AX
00°
mm
A
6; F VECTRA
1995/10/23 16:17:44
Localizer Sag
@3D @FC
@HE @PJ
3
0
cm
R
H01
0.50T
TOF(25°)
TR: 60
TI: 0
TE: 10
ECHO: 1/ 1
FOV:19cm
NEX: 1
MAT:128H/224V
06min08sec
L
P
WW354 WL+384
E.U. TIP FAK RADYODIAGNOST

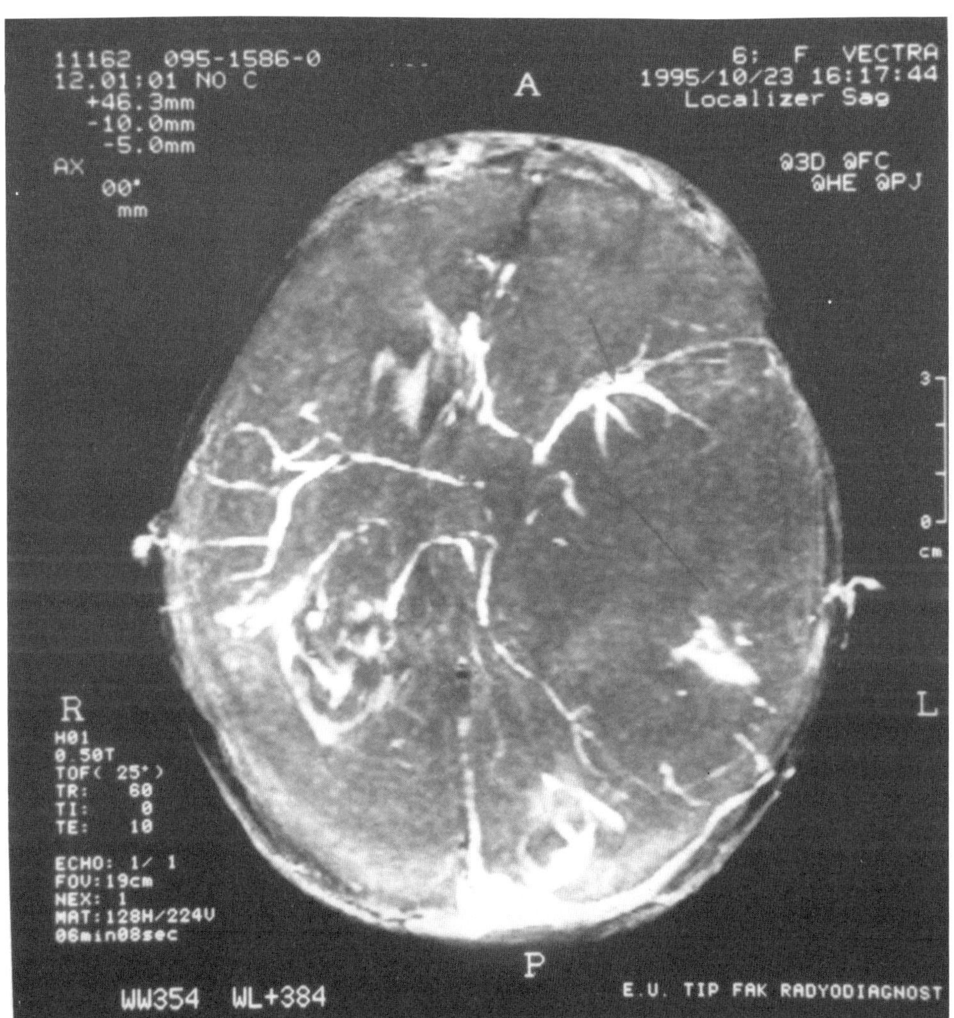

40g

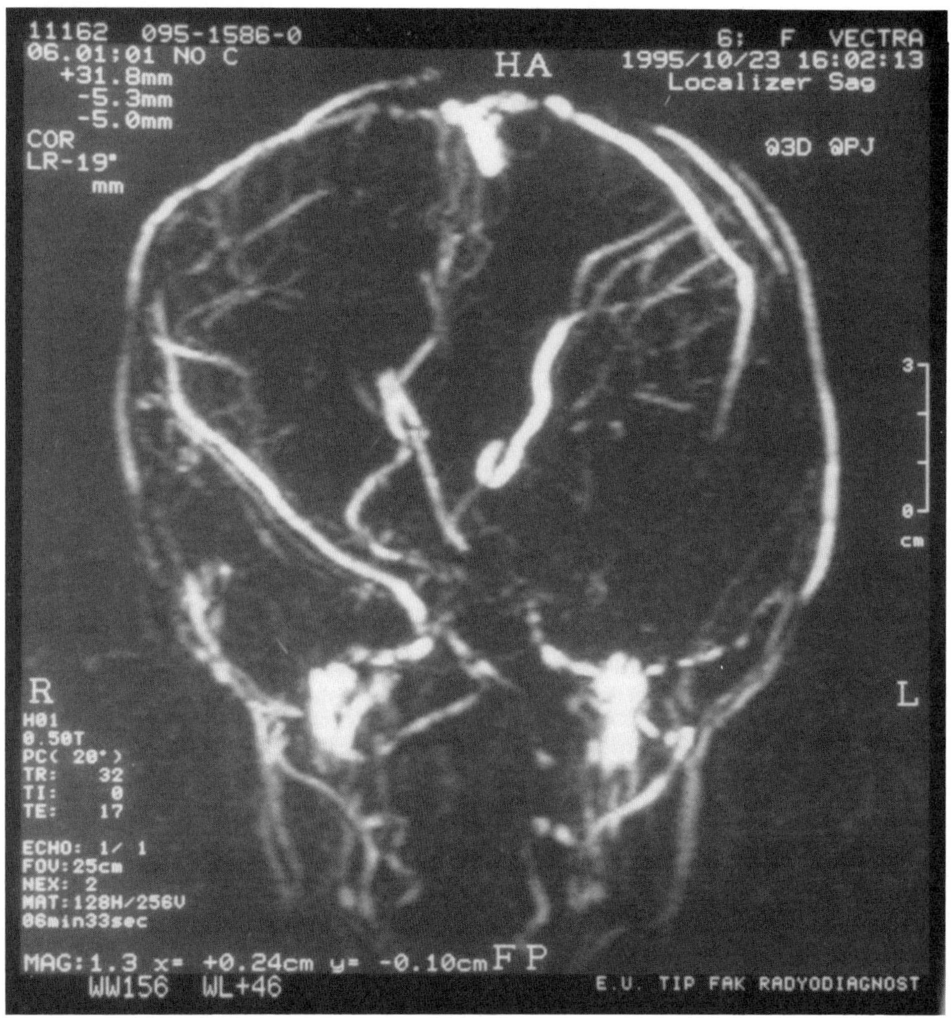

40h

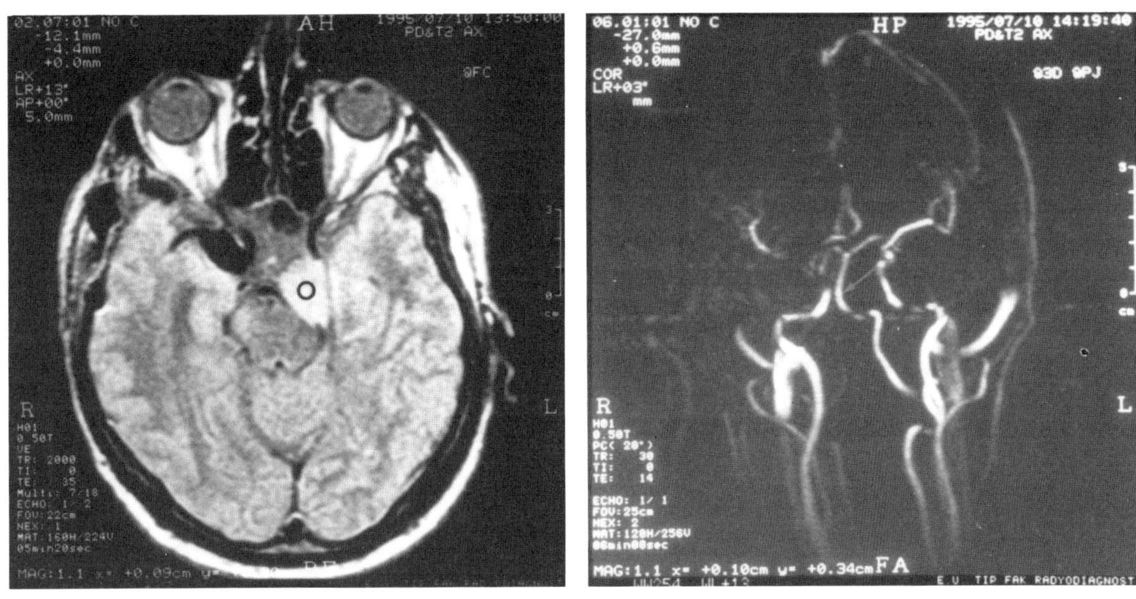

41a   41b

Fig. 41 *a,b. Meningioma of the clivus causing vascular displacement.* Adult patient.
a, axial PDW, and *b,* 3D-PC MRA. A meningioma originating from the left clivus (circle,
a) causes a compression upon the pons, and displaces the basilar artery (arrow, *b*).

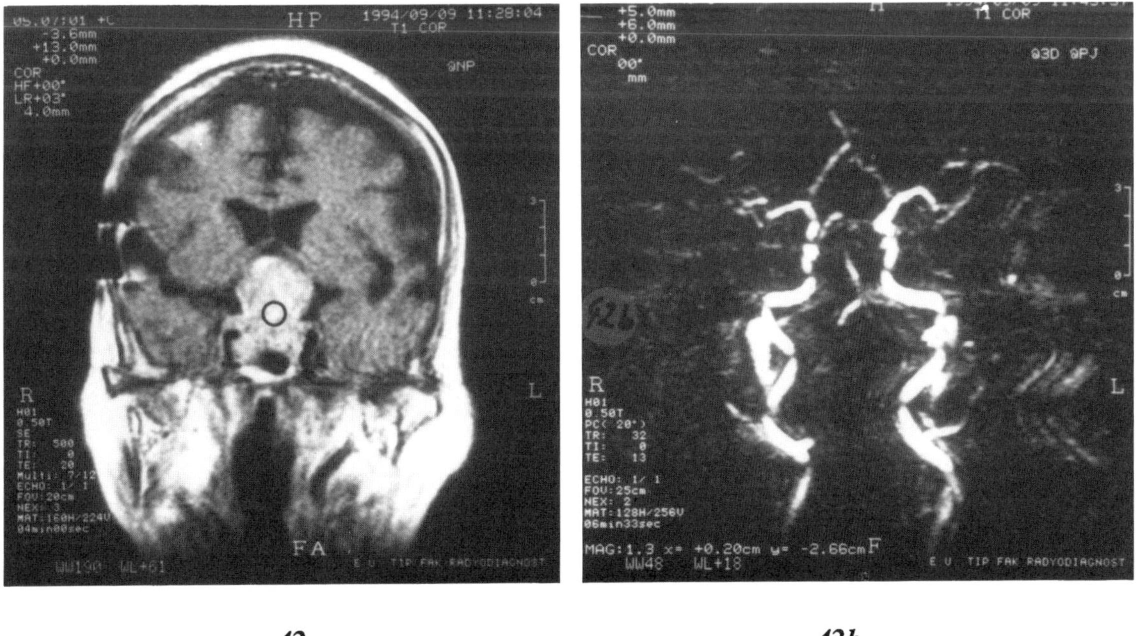

42a   42b

Fig. 42 *a,b. Adenoma of the hypophysis causing vascular displacement.* Adult patient.
a, axial T1W after administration of contrast-medium, and *b,* 3D-PC MRA. A large adenoma
(circle, *a*), displaces the internal carotid (short arrows), and middle cerebral (long arrows)
arteries (*b*).

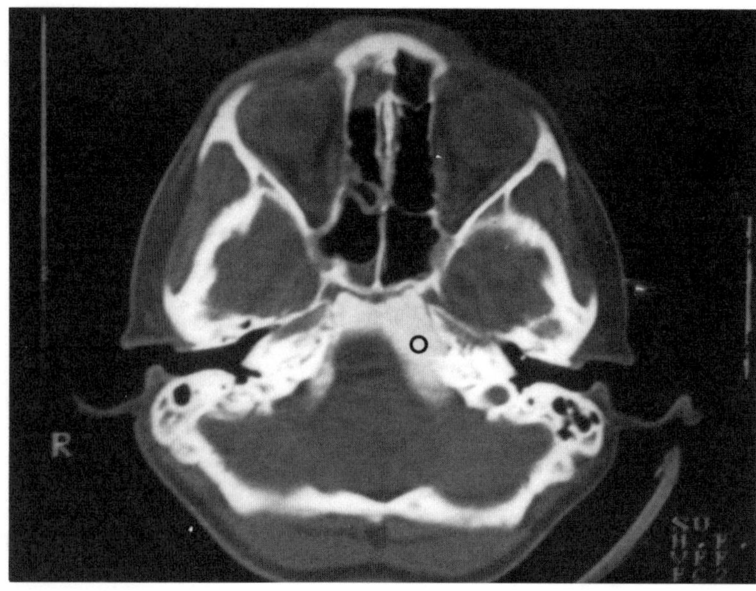

43a

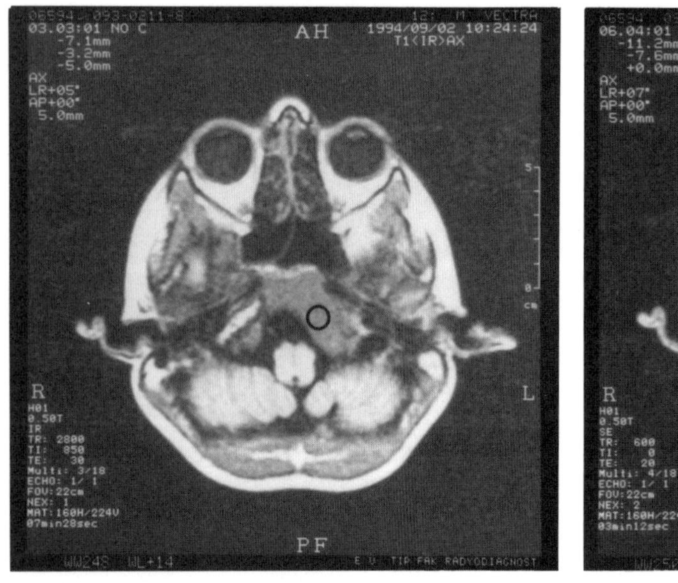

43b

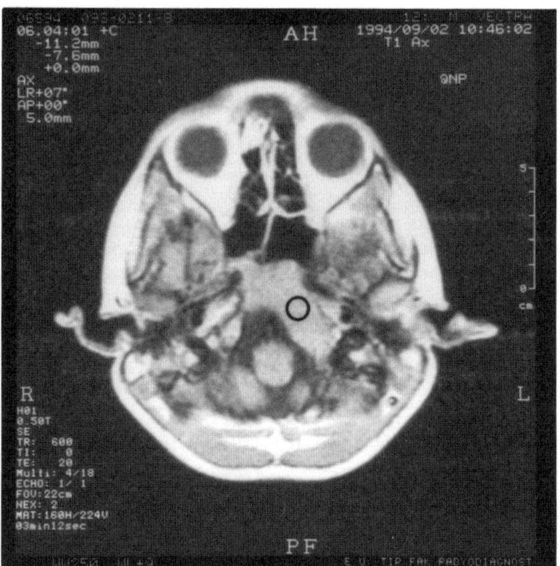

43c

Fig. 43 *a-e*. *Fibrous dysplasia of the clivus causing vascular displacement.* 12-year-old boy. *a,* CT scan; *b,* T1W (inversion recovery); *c,* T1W after administration of contrast-medium; *d,* T2W, and *e,* 3D-PC MRA. CT scan shows that the left part of the clivus is sclerotic, and enlarged (circle, *a*). The lesion (circles, *b-d*) gives low signal on the T2W image (*d*), compared with the T1W image (*b*), and shows an increased signal after administration of contrast-medium (*c*) compared with the T1W image (*b*). This is consistent with fibrous dysplasia. 3D-PC MRA shows displacement of the left vertebral artery (arrow, *e*).

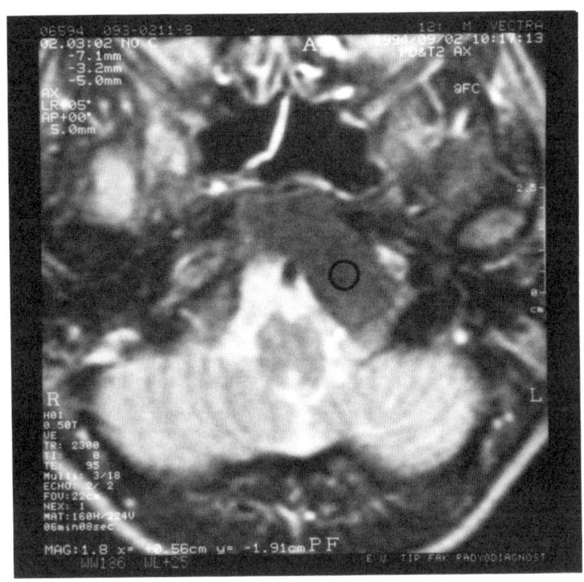

43d

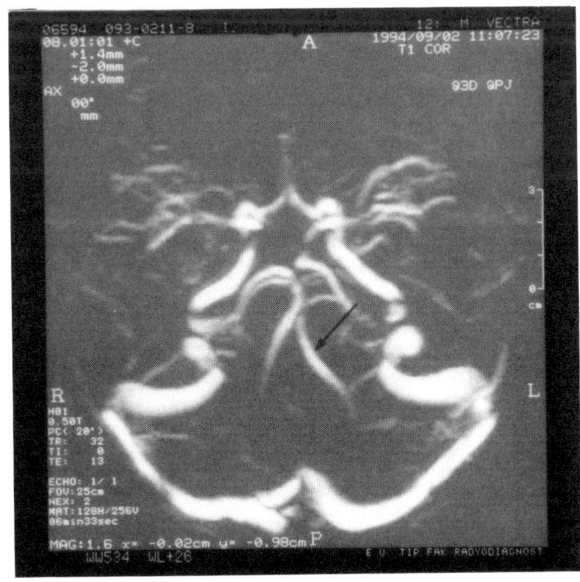

43e

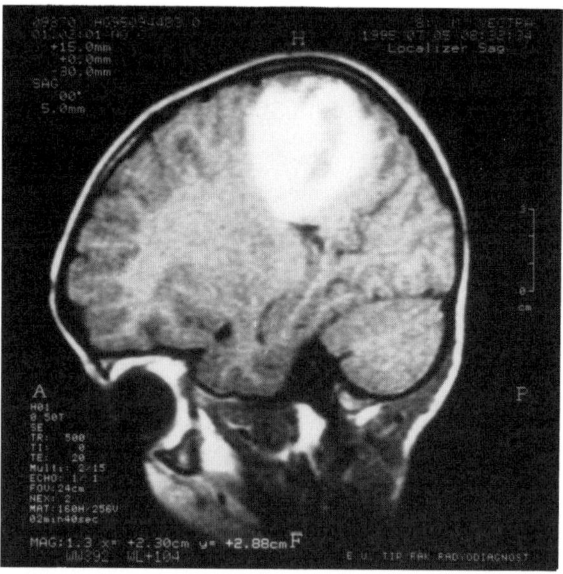

44a

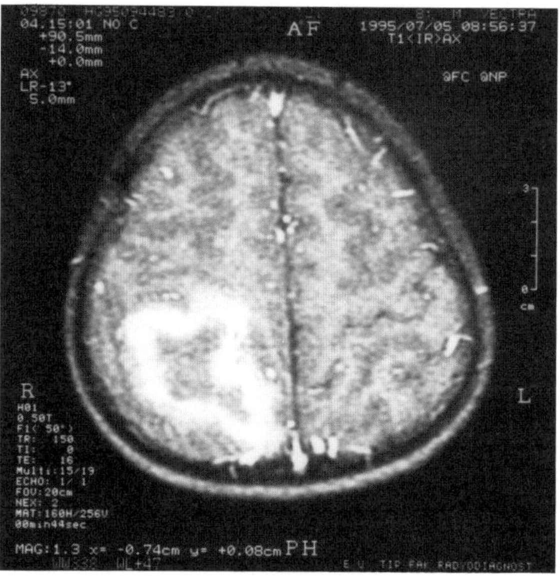

44b

Fig. 44 *a-g. Intracerebral hemorrhage.* 8-year-old boy. *a,* sagittal T1W; *b,* axial GRE T1W; *c,* axial T2W; *d,* axial 3D-TOF MRA; *e,* sagittal 3D-TOF MRA; *f,* coronal 3D-PC MRA, and *g,* sagittal 3D-PC MRA. There is mass with an hyperintense rim, and a relatively hypointense intense core on the T1W (*a,b*), and T2W (*c*) images. The rim represents extracellular methemoglobin, while the core represents intracellular methemoglobin of the subacute phase of intracerebral hemorrhage. In addition, the T2W image shows surrounding

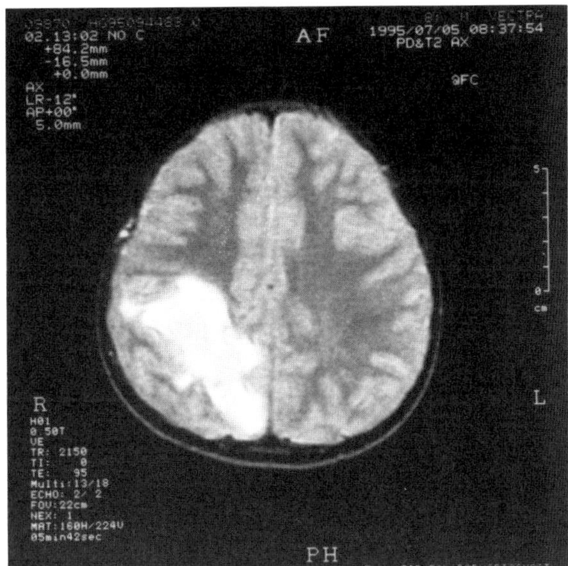

44c

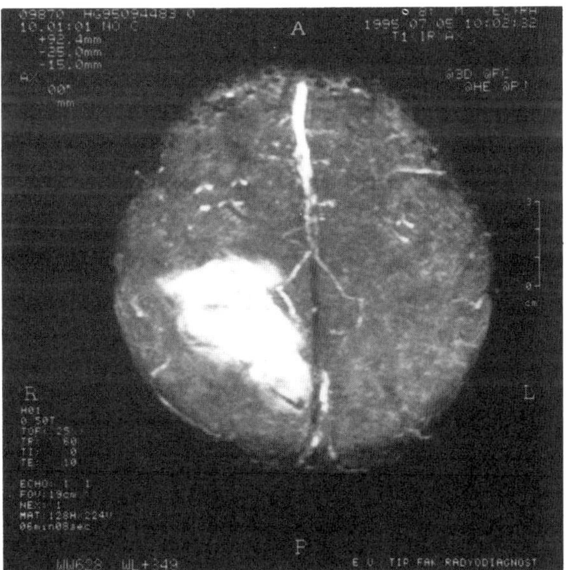

44d

high-signal edema (*c*). MR angiography was performed to exclude an underlying vascular lesion in this patient with hemorrhagic diathesis of unknown cause. The MIP reconstructions of the 3D-TOF MRA show the hemorrhagic region with high-signal, therefore they are not useful (*d,e*). However, the 3D-PC MRA with its excellent background suppression, demonstrates that there is no underlying vascular lesion (*f, g*) (see Fig 5) A conventional angiography was negative for a vascular lesion.

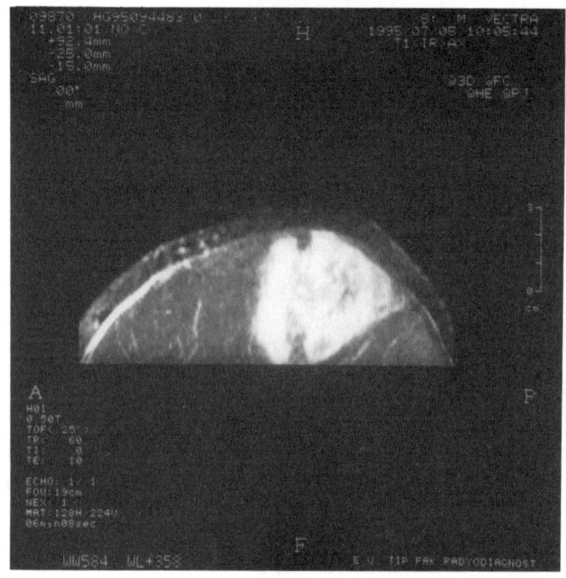

44e

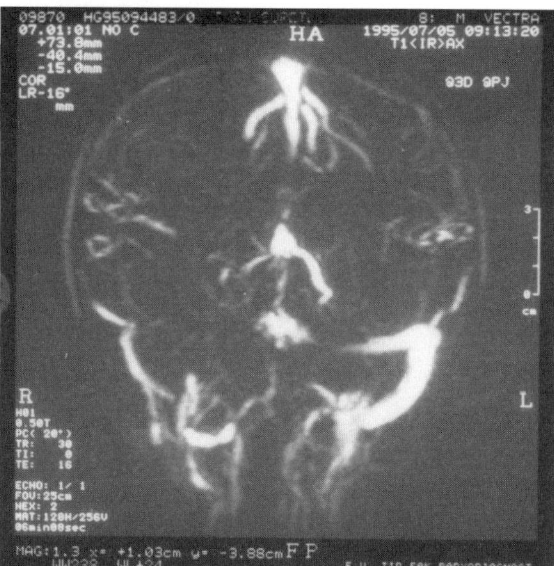

44f

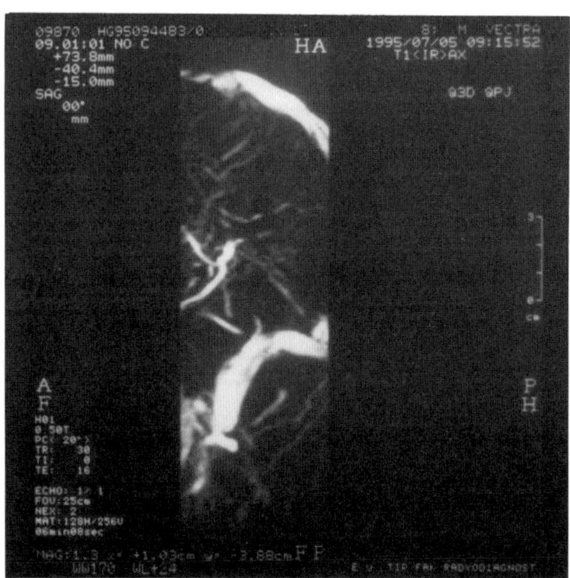

44g

REFERENCES

1. ApSimon, H.T., Ives, F.J., & Khangure, M.S. (1993) Cranial dural arteriovenous malformation and fistula. Radiological diagnosis and management. Review of thirty four patients. *Australas Radiol 37:2-25*.

2. Araki, Y., Kohmura, E., & Tsukaguchi, I. (1994) A pitfall in detection of intracranial unruptured aneurysms on three-dimensional phase-contrast MR angiography. *AJNR 15:1618-1623*.

3. Barkovich, A.J. (1995) Pediatric neuroimaging. Raven Press, New York.

4. Barkovich, A.J. (1988) Abnormal vascular drainage in anomalies of neuronal migration. *AJNR 9:939-942*.

5. Bowen, B.C., et al. (1994) MR angiography of occlusive disease of the arteries in the head and neck: current concepts. *AJR 162:9-18*.

6. Bui, L.N., et al. (1993) Magnetic resonance angiography of cervicocranial dissection. *Stroke 24:126-131*.

7. Chakeres, D.W., et al. (1991) Normal venous anatomy of the brain: demonstration with gadopentetate dimeglumine in enhanced 3-D MR angiography. *AJNR 11:1107-1118*.

8. Chen, J.C., Tsuruda, J.S., & Halbach, V.V. (1992) Suspected dural arteriovenous fistula: results with screening MR angiography in seven patients. *Radiology 183:265-271*.

9. Creasy, J.L., et al. (1990) Gadolinium-enhanced MR angiography. *Radiology 175:280-283*.

10. Damiano, T.R., et al. (1994) Posterior fossa venous angiomas with drainage through the brain stem. *AJNR 15:643-652*.

11. Davis, W.L., et al. (1994) Intracranial MR angiography: comparison of single-volume three-dimensional time-of-flight and multiple overlapping thin slab acquisition techniques. *AJR 163:915-920*.

12. Dumoulin, C.L., et al. (1989) Three-dimensional phase contrast angiography. *Magn Reson Med 9:139-149*.

13. Fujita N., et al. (1994) MR imaging of middle cerebral artery stenosis and occlusion: value of MR angiography. *AJNR 15:335-341*.

14. Gomori, J.M., et al. (1986) Occult cerebral vascular malformations: high-field MR imaging. *Radiology 158:707-713.*

15. Greenan, T.J., Grossman, R.I., & Goldberg, H. I. (1992) Cerebral vasculitis: MR imaging and angiographic correlation. *Radiology 182:65-72.*

16. Harris, K.G., et al. (1994) Diagnosing intracranial vasculitis: the roles of MR and angiography. *AJNR 15:317-330.*

17. Huston, J., III, and Ehman, R. L. (1993) Comparison of time-of-flight and phase-contrast MR neuroangiographic techniques. *Radiographics 13:5-19.*

18. Huston J., III, et al. (1994) Blinded prospective evaluation of sensitivity of MR angiography to known intracranial aneurysms: importance of aneurysm size. *AJNR 15:1607-1614.*

19. Huston J., III, et al. (1991) Intracranial aneurysms and vascular malformations: comparison of time-of-flight and phase-contrast MR angiography. *Radiology 181:721-730.*

20. Klufas, R.A., et al. (1995) Dissection of the carotid and vertebral arteries: imaging with MR angiography. *AJR 164:673-677.*

21. Lasjaunias, P., et al. (1991) Deep venous drainage in great cerebral vein (vein of Galen) absence and malformations. *Neuroradiology 33:234-238.*

22. Leonard, K., and Mamourian, A. C. (1989) MR appearance of intracranial chloromas. *AJNR (suppl) 10:67-68.*

23. Lewin, J.S., and Laub, G. (1991) Intracranial MR angiography: a direct comparison of three time-of-flight techniques. *AJNR 12:1133-1139.*

24. Mattle, H.P., et al. (1991) Cerebral venography with MR. *Radiology 178:453-458.*

25. Nussel, F., Wegmuller, H., & Huber, P. (1991) Comparison of magnetic resonance angiography, magnetic resonance imaging and conventional angiography in cerebral arteriovenous malformation. *Neuroradiology 33:56-61.*

26. Osborn, A.G. (1994) Diagnostic neuroimaging. Mosby, St. Louis.

27. Ostertun, B., and Solymosi, L. (1993) Magnetic resonance angiography of cerebral developmental venous anomalies: its role in differential diagnosis. *Neuroradiology 35:97-104.*

28. Robertson, S.J., Wolpert, S.M., & Runge, V.M. (1989) MR imaging of middle cranial fossa arachnoid cysts: temporal lobe agenesis syndrome revisited. *AJNR 10:1007-1010.*

29. Ross, J. S., et al. (1990) Intracranial aneurysms: evaluation by MR angiography. *AJR 155:159-165.*

30. Seidenwurm, D., et al. (1991) Vein of Galen malformation: correlation of clinical presentation, arteriography, and MR imaging. *AJNR 12:347-354.*

31. Sener, R.N. (1995) MR angiography of abnormal vascular structures in polymicrogyria. *IMIR (International Medical Image Registry) 1:43-44.*

32. Sener, R.N. (1995) MR angiographic demonstration of leukemic vasculopathy involving the middle cerebral arteries. *IMIR (International Medical Image Registry) 1:65-66.*

33. Sener, R.N. (1997) MR angiography of the vein of Galen Malformation. *Clinical Imaging* (in press).

34. Sener, R.N. (1995) Abnormal venous drainage in periventricular leukomalacia: an MR angiographic study. *Comput Med Imag Graph 19: 495-499.*

35. Sener, R.N. (1997) An extensive type of polyostotic fibrous dysplasia. *Pediatric Radiology* (in press).

36. Shoemaker, E.I., et al. (1994) Primary angiitis of the central nervous system: unusual MR appearance. *AJNR 331-334.*

37. Sze, G., et al. (1989) MR imaging of the cranial meninges with emphasis on contrast enhancement and meningeal carcinomatosis. *AJR 153:1039-1043.*

38. Truwit, C.L., et al. (1992) Cerebral palsy: MR findings in 40 patients. *AJNR 13:67-78.*

39. Vogl, T. J., et al. (1994) Dural sinus thrombosis: value of venous MR angiography for diagnosis and follow-up. *AJR 162:1191-1198.*

40. Vogl, T. J., et al. (1993) MR and MR angiography of Sturge-Weber syndrome. *AJNR 14:417-425.*

41. Wolpert, S.M., and Barnes, P.D. (1992) MRI in pediatric neuroradiology. Mosby Year Book, St. Louis.

42. Yamada, I., Matsushima, Y., & Suzuki, S. (1992) Moyamoya disease: diagnosis with three-dimensional time-of-flight MR angiography. *Radiology 184:773-778.*

Index

ABOUT THE AUTHOR

R. Nuri Sener, M.D., born in 1953, serves as the Chief of the Pediatric Radiology and Neuroradiology sections and of the Magnetic Resonance unit at the Department of Radiology of Ege University, Izmir, Turkey, where he holds the position of Professor of Radiology. He completed a Neuroradiology research fellowship between 1990 and 1991 at the Neuroradiology section of the University of Texas, Health Science Center at San Antonio, Texas, USA. Dr. Sener's primary field of research is Pediatric Neuroradiology. Dr. Sener has served as a visiting Professor at the Radiology Department in the Ullevaal Hospital of Oslo University, Oslo, Norway, the Royal Alexandra Hospital for Children, Sydney, Australia, and the Hospital of Sao Paulo University, Sao Paulo, Brazil.